CIGARETTE SEDUCTION

THE SECRET CODE TO QUITTING
FOR TOBACCO & E-CIGARETTE PRODUCTS

What You Smoked is How You Quit

By Alan Brody

e-Cigarettes and Cigarette Seduction

Welcome to the e-Cigarette version of **Cigarette Seduction**. While this book's only mission is to decode smoking and not take sides, it goes without saying that we would prefer that people were healthy.

With this book, you will understand what got you into smoking and why your brand has a mystical hold over you. That could either help you quit, ennoble you as a smoker or give you a new kind of tool to understand your colleagues and loved ones.

That's all good, but the biggest thing to happen to smoking in the past 10 years is the invention of the Electronic Cigarette or e-Cigarette. In many ways, this book is the training wheels for a world that will inevitably have to deal with this reconstructed smoking phenomenon: you cannot deconstruct the cigarette without also deconstructing the brands that made the habit so successful!

We want people to try e-Cigarettes because they are a wonderful first step in quitting. While some people may use them as a smoking alternative because they are arguably safer, cheaper, have no smell and little stigma they are really a step into the new world of smoking.

From our perspective they look and largely feel, like cigarettes yet they break some of the key elements that tie smokers to tobacco. By being artificial, they lose some of the tactile sensation that gives smoking its sensual attraction. The vapor may be a great substitute for smoke but it lacks the intoxication of real fumes so that moving to e-Cigarettes is the first step in breaking the chain of tobacco addiction.

e-Cigarettes are also the first blast in a new kind of war between drug purveyors that will underlines the true calculus of smoking: since smoking addresses certain hard-to-comprehend human needs, it really has not gone away. Where smoking has been reduced, the underlying need has probably shifted to other outlets - mostly prescription drugs. This is the zero sum game of cessation. As we will argue – it is better to manage this revolution than to ban it.

In any case, e-Cigarettes are a minor technological marvel. Conceptually, they are a deconstructed cigarette that uses electronics to deliver flavored nicotine in a kind of benign, flavored haze. Whether you use this as an alternative or as a first step in quitting, the net result is you can begin untangling the lure of smoking.

Unlike most quitting programs, we do not think of smoke cessation as one battle. We see it as two: is a mental as well as a physical proposition - and we do not recommend confronting both at the same time. In many ways, the physical addiction to nicotine and the oral aspects of smoking are relatively easy to overcome – it is the deep psychic attachment that is the hardest and very few cessation programs address that with any depth.

For many who are deeply bound to smoking, we think they should move the habit to an unfamiliar place, break the elements apart and solve them separately. So, while you are still "smoking" in a different form, you can begin to tackle the mental process, developing the kinds of strategies we describe in **Cigarette Seduction**.

In the meantime, by "vaping", you will stop reeking of tobacco, you will feel your lungs somehow clearing, your stamina might begin to return, you won't have to step into the freezing cold to indulge your habit and you will save a lot of money to boot.

We wish you or your loved one the best in quitting, knowing that this is a great first step. Most of all - even if they cannot quit, they and everyone around them will be the better for this smoking alternative.

Either way – whether eCigarettes are a waystation to quitting or an alternate lifestyle, **Cigarette Seduction** tells you who you really are by what you smoke.

About this Book
*The Big Lie – the Really Big Lie – is that smoking is all about addiction. **The Really Big Lie is** that some poor vulnerable teen was drawn in by advertising or peer pressure, got hooked and **then** just can't kick the habit.*
The truth is so much more complex but also simpler: For one thing – and new research on the brain proves this – once you no longer find personal value in

smoking, the addiction almost instantly vanishes. ("Brain Injury Disrupts Smoking Addiction" Science, Jan. 2007

For another thing, smokers are more fully aware than non-smokers of the dangers of smoking. And it is not that non-smokers are in denial – it is that the personal mystique, the internal magic of smoking – feels more powerful than its potential to wreck their health. There is also research showing that smokers are 3 times more likely than non-smokers to be depressed. Many others have suffered from the effect of some type of psychopathology.

You can use the code of your cigarette brands to understand the source of your smoking so that can resolve these issues or learn to replace smoking with other, healthier practices.

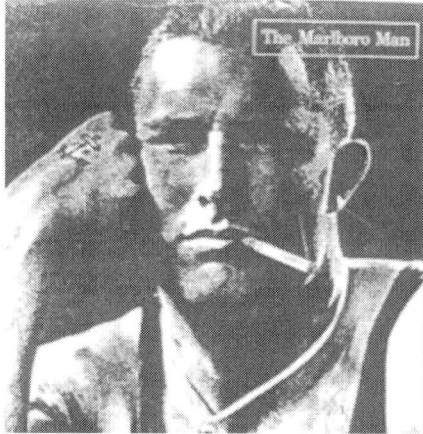

In Cigarette Seduction, we peel back the layers of meaning that have become attached to this 20th Century product and not only help you quit, but help you "unsmoke" so that you will never have the need to smoke again. Ever.

Best of all, many of the sources of this book are the tobacco industry itself. The tobacco industry has been doing research on this product at a deeper level for a lot longer than you ever imagined. I studied these now forgotten sources and even became the disciple of one its pioneers, the late Dr. Ernest Dichter. Using a combination of the industry's work with a growing body of research in non-verbal communication and neuroscience, this book will take you into the heart of smoking to enable you to imagine your life without it and escape it, becoming a better person

Cigarette Seduction *will show you how deep smoking really is and then unlock the code that makes it work on you!*

PROLOG

How Cigarette Brands Work on Teen and Adult Smokers is the critical element in understanding the way to quit. Your brand history is the key to making this work for you.

If there is one thing you need to know about cigarettes it is this: cigarettes are the "crack" of tobacco products. The power of this form of "crack" is not as much in its addiction or its faint, mind-altering powers. The power lies in its combination of inhalation and the age when you started – e.g., in your teens –

which turns this into a profound personality prop that makes it extremely difficult for you to quit when you grow up.

Smoking may be hundreds, even thousands **of** years old. But cigarettes were only developed in the mid-19th Century with a new kind of low-cost inhalable tobacco called *Bright*. Prior to that, smoking was a foul-smelling, mostly male practice that involved coarse tobaccos that could not be inhaled.

With the invention of mass-production machines, cigarettes became widely available but were considered effete, until they were popularized by **World War I** soldiers. The fact that they were new kind of phenomenon that could appeal to men and women and could be inhaled without the dense smell associated with cigars, attracted new kinds of hucksters - and researchers.

Instead of users spitting out chew tobacco or fouling the air with cigars or aromatic pipes, these immensely portable and highly penetrating, low-cost items could be sold to just about anyone to be consumed just about anywhere. Advertising gave them personality, society endorsed them, and many ancient rituals attached themselves to this new kind of deep breathing exercise.

None of this was lost on the pioneering marketers of smoke. Since the 1920s, tobacco companies have been on a quest to understand why people smoke. Starting with Sigmund Freud's nephew, E.L Bernays, who helped American Tobacco introduce Lucky Strike to new generations of smokers, tobacco companies have infused cigarettes with knowledge drawn from psychoanalysis.

In the 1950s, a new generation of brands was launched, with Marlboro at the forefront. With the guidance of psychological motivation researchers like Ernest Dichter, who became this author's mentor, cigarettes have evolved into much more than a simple habit: they are a way of life that began partly as initiation into adulthood, **party as a** status symbol, **partly as** self-medication, and **partly as a** mythic quest to evolve one's self.

The Secret of Quitting Revealed – By You

If you have been trying to quit – and discovered the abyss you face – this is the only book that will help you discover your passage out of it.

Only you know why you really started and only you know how to really quit. But first you need to decode the message of your brand and the part it plays in your psyche. Then, quitting is just like relearning a familiar skill.

Cigarette Seduction shows the "secret language" of cigarettes and how you have formed a lifetime of attachments to them. Once you understand how this works, you will feel like you have the keys to your salvation - and a new sense of wisdom.

If you are in a hurry to quit, go directly to chapters 10-14 so you can understand how to decode your brand, soul search your smoking motivation, and develop a sound quitting strategy and closure ceremony. You may be one of the lucky few who can quit spontaneously. Most people can't because smoking has taken on a deep, unwitting significance in their lives.

You need to know a lot more about cigarettes to understand how they assumed a pivotal role in your life. You will need to grasp how cigarettes became an accepted part of the culture and your lifestyle, because you will have to fill all those gaps in your post-smoking life. Otherwise, you will be irresistibly drawn back to smoking like a bungee cord.

Recidivism is the fate of most quitters because they underestimate the role of cigarettes in their lives. Cigarette Seduction shows how cigarette smoking grew as a cultural and spiritual force that has entered your life. It gives you the tools and the profound technique to overcome it, because once you know what your cigarettes really stand for and how you can release them, you can quit. You just need the motivation......and the deep story of smoking may provide that for you.

This book will show what smoking is really all about – first, from the view of savvy tobacco company researchers and then in terms borne out by the recent research of neuroscientists. In addition, we have gathered profiles from hundreds of smokers in the United States, Canada and the United Kingdom, and we provide a description of the leading brands' perceived meaning and "inner traits."

At the end of this book we provide an appendix with sample profiles that show how teens initiate within a web of peer and familial influence. We see them find their own brand in reaction to that brand's perceived meaning and then watch how their brand choices evolve as their lives change until they reach middle age.

Background

People first became aware of the real importance of cigarette marketing - negative as it was - in 1988, when it became possible to put a monetary value on smoking. That was when a New Jersey court awarded the late Rose Cipollone's estate $400,000 from the Lorillard tobacco company because it found that the company had persuaded her to smoke through its marketing. For the first time, a relationship between smoking and cigarette ads had been established as a legal reality with a dollar value attached.

As it turns out, the award was only a temporary setback for the industry because the wording of the health warnings on the cigarette packs enabled a higher court to overturn the award. The health warning labels were upheld as a reasonable warning to smokers about the dangers of the product. Still, Cipollone's estate proved that she was lured by those ads prior to 1966 when the warning labels first appeared. And even though the victory was fleeting, people got the point: the advertising and marketing of tobacco is worth something. It has some effect on getting people to smoke and it seems to keep them smoking. Even now, the government and an array of lawyers continue to attack the industry with generally limited success beyond the great tobacco settlement of 1997, when Big Tobacco agreed to pay up $25 billion a year in a historic deal. The industry agreed to pay $368 billion in health-related damages, tear down billboards, and retire Joe Camel.

Like so much in this industry, the settlement was not quite what it seemed. It really wasn't the tobacco companies that paid for it - it was the smokers who paid with the drastic increase in the price of cigarettes. As for the settlement money, most of it has gone into pork barrel and budget-balancing projects. Very little has gone into health issues. (See "Where Has All the Tobacco Money Gone?" ABC News April 12, 2007 www.abc.go.com or my article in Newsday, Tobacco-Pact Money Is Misdirected," Newsday, Aug, 27, 2001, p. 18.)

Not all is at it seems with smoking either. While advertising and marketing have their role there is a lot more to smoking than simple persuasion. Society has its role but so do smokers. They were never entirely unaware of its dangers, and evidence shows that in many ways its riskiness was always part of the attraction. This is the dirty secret of quitting: you need to know how to deal with the negative feelings because they will not disappear, and without a strategy they will return to drag you back into smoking.

As the so-called habit of smoking came to be recognized as a true addiction, courts were more apt to buy the argument that people were lured into smoking - particularly in the late nineteen forties and early fifties when cigarette ads came with virtual promises of health benefits. Recently, a California court awarded the estate of a smoker $28 billion before appeal. It is worth remembering that this approach probably first began to work in 1996 when the Carter estate won their case against Brown & Williamson. Grady Carter was enticed by the cigarette advertising promises of the nineteen fifties and then became hopelessly addicted. One particularly compelling piece of testimony was a reel of TV ads that involved claims like "Not a Cough in a Carload" (Old Gold) "More Doctors Smoke Camel" and "No Throat Irritation" (Philip Morris).

Then, in the wake of the cancer scare, a series of highly publicized medical warnings in the early fifties, cigarette advertising became more subtly seductive and seemed to blend into the general media background. It was the revelation in the late nineteen eighties that RJ Reynolds had announced a new brand of cigarettes for African-Americans that aroused the ire of the new Health Secretary, Dr. Louis Sullivan. As the nation's chief doctor and an African-American whose people were being targeted by this unhealthy product, he made this a national issue. Then, just as commentators raised the point that cigarette companies had been doing that for years with women, compelling evidence emerged of a new kind of woman being targeted. A new breed of liberated blue collar woman had been singled out for product development, according to "internal documents" from a marketing company working for RJ Reynolds. This new evidence showed that indeed, women hadn't been forgotten. According to these leaked plans, the R.J. Reynolds company was getting ready to launch a new brand called Dakota, aimed at the virile, blue-collar female who had no more than a high school education, liked tractor pulls, boyfriends, and identified strongly with Roseanne, the hefty TV star. Now, in the first decade of the twenty first century, RJ Reynolds is doing the same thing with **Camel No. 9** for women.

The idea that cigarettes can actually be aimed at specific groups of people - in essence, fatally exploiting their weaknesses - shocked people. The tone of the press reports that covered the story seemed to suggest "*how could they?*" Yet marketing is marketing, and as long as cigarettes are a legal product why *shouldn't* people expect tobacco companies to behave the same way as soap marketers who target their customers by their personality profiles. Who cares if soap marketers have a fine understanding of the sexual and mythical underpinnings of cleaning - that washing with soap is a way of removing sin or controlling sexual desire. It is only soap. But with cigarettes it is different because of the disturbing thought that not only is tobacco dangerous but *what if the cigarettes really meant something?* What if the brands had meaning and a special value of their own so that they not only revealed the smoker but also represented a kind of mythological value system that no amount of reasoning or legislation can undermine?

Cigarette Seduction is about *what cigarettes really mean.* The insights are a way to inform us with an interpretive, psychological knowledge of the cigarette phenomenon and a vocabulary of ideas to deal with the issues of smoking. The book also follows the various marketing approaches taken by the majors when dealing with their public image: the leader, Philip Morris taking the "high road" and inculcating religion and national honor into their marketing plans, while the follower, RJ Reynolds, out of touch with the climate of non-smokers, temporarily succeeding with such transparently dangerous approaches as talking back to their critics and developing a cartoon Camel that attracts children - only to provoke society's consequent retribution.

Cigarette Seduction confronts the fundamental questions about this practice of smoking which is at once atavistic, dangerous, unexplained and widely practiced. This is a media-savvy investigation into the mystery of smoking the way it is: what smoking really means and how that information can be used to quit or simply to gain an understanding of the smokers' motivation in business or social life.

To begin with, this is not an anti-smoking treatise. This author is no fan of smoking, but the fact is that in life we are often asked to sacrifice long-term health for the ability to function well on a day-to-day basis. Take the example of Psychology Today. It has been an organ of the American Psychological Association and as such, a quasi-medical journal. Yet, unlike the typical health or medical journal, while it was a for-profit publication, it teemed with cigarette ads. While at one level that was purely mercenary, it also said that the mental health establishment tacitly supports smoking because cigarettes work as a kind of over-the-counter form of therapy. Was not Freud a great cigar lover, even while his cigars were killing him with throat cancer?

Realistically, a healthy body is a wonderful thing but it is worthless without a functioning mind, and that is where smoking retains its magic. People derive momentary power from smoking for a combination of reasons that go beyond imagination and physiology. This is in effect the modern face - the avatar - of an old way of ordering our lives: living according to a set of dream stories and archetypes that we ordinarily call mythology. With cigarettes, we can consume these myths in a form of branded smoke.

The mission of this book is to help you preserve a healthy state of mind, avoid judgment of your lapses, and lead you to a life of *unsmoking* – dealing with your life's issues the way you did before your learned to smoke.

To understand the flexible lure of smoking, one has only to consider the campaign RJ Reynolds launched after their cartoon Joe Camel was banished from their ads: a woman with a come-hither expression and tight, sexy clothing exhaling smoke embedded with the image of a Camel. *Smoke this, young man,* she is saying, *and you can have all that you lust for*. Young women who need to project this sultry image will fall for this too. It is in its own way a perfect summary of the state of cigarettes appeal: visible, in the form of an obvious seductress and reaching below consciousness as an embedded message understandable to anyone who has fallen for the idea of obnoxious fumes having the power to embolden them.

With its long history and recurring supply of converts, cigarettes are not going to disappear. The proportion of smokers in the population seems to be declining (except that is, for women) but the absolute numbers are almost unchanged over the past twenty years. Over 50 million people in this country continue to smoke. From an economic point of view, the tobacco industry is doing as well as or better than ever.

While opposition to smoking has become a virtual public policy, smoking continues. Despite all that damning and conclusive evidence against it, its continuing practice still remains an open mystery that both smokers and non-smokers have been unable to fathom.

Taking an unblinking look at human frailty flirts with the possibility of stepping into an abyss. Much of smoking's appeal, after all, is as compensation for life's shortcomings. People yearn for impossible things that are also often unmentionable. So, looking at both smoking and smokers in a true light dredges up some equally unmentionable things. You may learn some revealing lessons on how to read people from their brands. More significantly, you can to learn about quitting smoking at a much deeper level than is usually offered by smoke-stop programs which are plagued by recidivism due to,- among other reasons, their shallowness.

There is nothing wrong with most smoke-stop programs, whether they involve a patch or a gum or substitution system. I recommend them - as far as they go. The problem is, they don't go far enough; they deal only with the mechanical side of smoking. Even if they help wean you from nicotine addiction they still doesn't get the real issue of smoking, which is in your associative mind. Smokers have evolved a symbolic support system which requires them to reach out for a smoke at each metered moment when the physical expression of the addiction calls for. If you don't resolve this issue, your needy psyche will simply call out for the addiction to be resumed and you will be back where you started from – minus the healthy break you took.

With Cigarette Seduction, readers will discover a symbolic system, a kind of simple visual language underscoring the cigarette world that also tells us about our own world. In a milieu where graphics have gone from the decorative, or in other cases, a kind of preliterate pidgin, to the highly informative language of mass marketing and even the visual interface of high technology, this study is eye-opening. The revelation of smoking is that it is an intensified world of visual cues where smokers have put their health at risk for the symbolic rewards of cigarettes.

Smokers who intend to remain in the fold will smoke a little more knowingly once they realize that their Marlboro is a thinly disguised military award. And for those who don't want to smoke at all, they will find ammunition

to quit once they understand what symbolic, if bogus, rewards America's top brands offer the public. To those tracking the tobacco industry, it is an inside look at the dialog the cigarette manufacturers have with their public. For the rest of us, this is a road map of the cigarette ethos and the way in which the industry tries to perpetuate its hold on the American psyche in the twenty-first century.

CIGARETTE SEDUCTION List of Chapters

INTRODUCTION:

SMOKING AS THE INITIATION RITUAL OF INDUSTRIAL SOCIETY

1).. **THE   MYTHIC SEDUCTION OF SMOKING**

.... In the deep background of smoking, two forgotten common ceremonies of primitive cultures lurk: initiation and mass trances. How they have continued, in a disguised form, are two of the most compelling reasons why so many people smoke.

2) .... **CAMEL: HOW   THE MYTH WAS FIRST BROUGHT TO MARKET**

....It took several years before tobacco companies discovered **this** myth. They seem to have discovered it by mistake and it wasn't until the **nineteen** twenties before anyone got around to psychoanalyzing it. But once they understood it they never let go. A look around the world shows that Madison Avenue wasn't the only place that knew a myth when it saw one. The French government did and the British fared rather well too.

3).. **THE PSYCHOLOGICAL EDGE OF SMOKING: PEOPLE THINK IT GIVES THEM A PERSONAL SENSE OF CONTROL**

.... An unblinking look at the great modern enigma: If smoking is deadly, and everyone knows it, why do we keep on doing it? We keep on doing it because it's a primal sense of self-control.

4).. **ORIGIN   OF   THE CIGARETTE**

.... Like everything else in life, cigarettes have a history. Except this is an interesting history that reveals a few cultural milestones in ways that we never quite saw them before.

5)   **DEATH AND SEX AND CIGARETTES**

Cigarettes are meaningful because they address the two things we can't live without.

6).. **HOW   MARLBORO BECAME A MAN.**

.... Marlboro didn't just get that way. First it had to go through a sex-change, find the right symbol, and, ultimately, the right myth. But with over 70 per cent of white high school students starting out smoking Marlboro, there has to be something more to this than meets the eye. In this case, that something is teenagers recognizing it as an initiation ritual.

7)   **THE CIGARETTE LANGUAGE**

Now that you have read the method, how do you make an interpretation in simple, common sense terms?

8)   **....AND WHAT KIND OF MAN?**

Now we know why people start smoking, what do the brands reveal about people who stay with them? Exactly what?
9)

THE I-QUITTING CHAPTERS

10)   THE MEANING OF THE MAJOR BRANDS
Applying the **Cigarette Seduction** theory of meaning to the most common major and generic brands available in America.
11)   READING THE SMOKER'S PERSONAL MYTHOLOGY
If you carry a cross in life then your brands will reflect it. This is how you find out what it is.
12)   USING YOUR BRANDS TO QUIT – FOR GOOD
What you smoke is also the roadmap to how to you quit.
13)   WELCOME TO THE NEW WORLD OF SMOKE
What happens when we evolve our understanding of smoking as self-medication and wealthy tobacco companies begin to evolve their quasi-medical relationship with consumers.
14)   e-CIGARETTES
Why e-Cigarettes will change everything.

Introduction: People Begin Smoking as a Tribal Ritual
When this author began smoking as a teenager, it was with one eye on an older culture in the background. I grew up in Africa in the southern reaches of

Zululand, now Kwazulu-Natal, where ancient rites of stick and spear fighting, and initiation and sorcery could still be observed on the edges of society. My induction into smoking took place just like most other people's - with a feeling of guilt for once making fun of adults who smoked and a feeling of defiance for having taken on something so obviously dangerous.

There was also a sense of inevitability to this, and my desire to smoke was something larger than myself. And as much as it was impossible to handle the desire at an intellectual level, it was also clear that as a teenager, I possessed a longing for some kind of initiation - a manifest, ritualized process that would guide me from youth to adulthood. For reasons not fathomable to me at the time, smoking seemed to offer a solution to that.

As a white middle class teenager in a faraway place, my path to adulthood followed the typical patterns of western society: music, popular culture, school, a profession. On the other side of the tracks, however, away from our west-ernized middle class side of town, the indigenous Africans still lived out the old culture where tribal gatherings and ritualized initiation ceremonies were an ongoing occurrence that gave its adherents a sense of order in life.

In reality, as Westerners, we were missing something. There would be no comparable ceremony to look forward to - no dramatic initiation test, no ac-ceptance, and no permanent symbol of recognition. Instead, we had that first puff. Yet, somehow, those scenes played out along the grassy roadsides of less-traveled highways - the ritual beatings of initiates at open-air church groups or the stickfights between rival groups of shield-carrying warriors seemed to have some kind of relationship to this unexplainable act of smoking.

During my college studies in the United States, my interest in advertising led to a simple observation: after World War II, the typical approach to advertising - getting the client's name before the public and putting his best foot forward - began to give way to a more sophisticated approach. Advertising had come to be understood as a business of selling products by interpreting the culture and establishing the status values of the products advertisers offered the public.

David Ogilvy, the phenomenally successful post-war advertising pioneer and British expatriate, considered ad people from other cultures as having a special advantage because they could bring an objective eye to the business. That certainly was my experience, and in studying the basic books by the industry's immortals - Hopkins, Ogilvy, Caples and Reeves - it was clear that while advertising at one level *is* that conventional portrait of how to put a product's best foot forward, creating a positive image and generally accentuating the positive, there was another side to it. While my experiences of growing up in post-colonial Africa initially seemed alien in the First World, that view changed abruptly after studying Vance Packard's **Hidden Persuaders** and the books by the advertising researchers he had interviewed in the nineteen fifties, including Ernest Dichter, Louis Cheskin, and Pierre Martineau, who had revolutionized post-World War II marketing. It became clear to me that the experience of primitive Africa matched the fifties exploitation of the id that was afoot on Madison Avenue during that time.

To a general audience during the McCarthy era of the fifties, the theme of Vance Packard's **Hidden Persuaders** perfectly matched the paranoia of the times. But there was so much more to the book than a simple exposé. What Packard described was really the emergence of a language of perceptions.

In many respects, Packard's book became a kind of Rosetta Stone of modern marketing, not just for what it said, but also for what it didn't say. Like the dog that didn't bark in the night in the Sherlock Holmes story of the **Hound of the Baskervilles**, the **Hidden Persuaders** had very little to say about the one product that is most dependent on psychological benefits: cigarettes. Guessing that the psychological underpinnings of smoking was a subject just too sensitive for an exposé of the fifties, I explored the work of all Packard's sources and found that two of them, Ernest Dichter and Louis Cheskin, had indeed worked for the tobacco companies. Dichter had even written a warning to the industry in the nineteen forties that they were "killing themselves" with the health massages in their ads, even publishing a study in 1947 entitled **Why We Smoke** (see p. 48). Cheskin had actually handled an important part of Marlboro's package research and even wrote a book about it entitled **How to Predict What People Will Buy**, featuring a picture of himself and the Marlboro project manager and future Chairman George Weissman.

To Ernest Dichter, one of the book's major characters, and the man who is widely regarded as the father of modern psychological research in advertising, the businessman proudly stepping out of his Rolls Royce is not that different from the African chief with his leopard skin, fly swish, and ceremonial feathers. Saying that the practices of American teenagers were as "fascinating a subject for investigation as the tribal customs and initiation rites of a primitive people," Dichter began, in the nineteen thirties with this mission of bringing cultural anthropology with a distinctly Freudian bent, first to Chrysler, CBS, and Proctor & Gamble, and then to Madison Avenue at large.

Dichter's professional career had been based on a connection I had made in an overlooked part of the world: we have status symbols just as primitive people do. The role of advertising in a consumer society is to discover what fills in for the status symbols and totemic objects that give our tribal counterparts their sense of identity and continuity. Where these objects tend to have a fixed role in primitive societies, they are almost always in flux in the modern world.

The irony is that the subject of tribal initiation has become an uncomfortable one in Africa; westerners tend to ignore the indigenous cultures and Africans prefer to be seen in a more modern light. So the idea of American businessmen or American youth borrowing from horrific rituals that often resulted in the scarring of initiates seemed uncertain at best. Yet smoking is not in any way a rational practice and, over time, enough outlandish hippies, skinheads, punks, Hell's Angels, and pierced and tattooed teens have emerged, demonstrating that initiation is a deep psycho-mythological need that youth will seek regardless of whether or not society can provide it for them.

The surprise was just how much of this had already been anticipated by Madison Avenue. The original Marlboro Man had been famous for tribal markings of his own - not for the tribal scars so common in Africa but rather, for an equivalent marking found among lighter-skinned people such as the Polynesians, nomadic Arabs, Japanese *yakuza,* and American Hell's Angels: the common tattoo. This is not a subject that marketing books or the memoirs of retired marketing executives have emphasized. But the real story is that Madison Avenue had taken a symbol directly from our tribal past and broadcast it over the media as a selling point. By now both Marlboro and its tattooed past have become so ingrained in the culture that it is pure marketing DNA and advertisers have been able to curtail their advertising without seriously risking their market penetration.

In ad schools the success of Marlboro is a standard case study. Marlboro is, far and away, the most successful cigarette brand of all time and today owns more than 25% of the U.S. market. The brand is usually described as a repackaging of a preexisting brand that came out in 1954. Its precursor, the original Marlboro, first appeared in the nineteen twenties and was sold to society ladies, with such slogans as "Marlboro. Mild as May" and, to emphasize its cardboard mouthpiece, "Ivory Tips Protect Your Lips." Then, along came George Weissman, a marketing wizard who recognized that in light of growing health concerns, a filtered cigarette could be made to sell if it had a certain brand personality. To achieve that, he took a failing woman's brand, repackaged and filtered it, and gave it a new, macho image. He also spent about $200,000 - a fantastic sum in nineteen fifties dollars - on various kinds of psychological and marketing research.

The success of Marlboro is legendary and it continues today. History records that Weissman went on to become Chairman of the giant Philip Morris corporation. Marketing books, however, rarely examine the nature of the research that propelled the **Marlboro** brand to the top. They never seem to ask just what Philip Morris was looking for in the package and why they chose to recycle a defunct brand - a rare practice in any market - when they could as easily have produced an entirely new one.

At the time, Philip Morris, like other tobacco companies, was merely responding to the public health scare by bringing out a filtered cigarette. Since filters were a new concept at that time, it follows that they should have brought out an entirely new brand. Yet even though the classic 1954 advertisement with a Marlon Brando look-alike sporting a tattooed anchor on his hand is commonly found in books on advertising, its anthropological significance is rarely discussed. Even the evolution of the cowboy is overlooked, and it is often forgotten that there were once Marlboro *men* - mechanics, lifeguards, detectives - and that it took several years before Philip Morris realized not just *any* macho man would do in their ads - it *had* to be a cowboy.

One of the people behind the packaging was Louis Cheskin, a researcher who appeared in Vance Packard's expose of the nineteen fifties "brainwashing" approach to advertising, **The Hidden Persuaders**. Cheskin's job was to test consumer response to the design by using such psychological testing devices as a pupillometer, to measure emotional response from the dilation of the viewer's pupil, an eye-tracking machine to examine what they looked *at* and afterwards, a tachistoscope to see what they noticed and remembered. According to Cheskin, the key element on the bright red Marlboro pack was the crest. Since the brand came out just as young GIs were returning from an unsatisfactory war in Korea, it is clear that Philip Morris was after something with a war motif. Something that would appeal to returning soldiers. Something that looked like a medal.

That explains why Marlboro has a bright red "ribbon" at the top of the box, a crest that resembles a medal and a slogan borrowed from Caesar at his most victorious: "Veni. Vidi. Vici. I came. I saw. I conquered." Philip Morris also took the risk of retaining the Marlboro name because it echoed the military title of Sir **Winston** Churchill's renowned ancestor, the Duke of Marlborough, a 17th Century general. Names of successful military leaders near times of war have a powerful resonance, roughly equivalent to the attention given General Colin Powell during the aftermath of the Gulf War.

Most authorities believe that cigarettes, which were once considered unmanly, first became popular as a result of World War I. Our soldiers picked up the habit from European soldiers in the trenches and cigarettes became part of the doughboys' rations. It seems obvious that two generations later a brilliant cigarette executive would find a marketing metaphor in war. More than that, it was Marlboro's special combination of elements that formed what is now recognizable as a myth: Marlboro is a hero's reward and as we know from the tattoo and the Western symbols that accompanied it, an enduring initiation symbol. By giving young soldiers returning from the unsatisfactory Korean war a cigarette pack with a phony medal on a stiff box, and using ads with tattoos, Marlboro went on to become Madison Avenue's greatest coup.

When marketing phenomena like these come under the microscope, advertising people generally evade scrutiny by harping on the old stereotype that Madison Avenue people are superficial and couldn't think that deeply if they tried. Often, that seems true because the bulk of an ad agency's work comprises mundane advertising work for brands that have little opportunity to distinguish themselves, and it takes many uninspired types to produce an ad. But those at the heart of the business - the ones who create the big, selling ideas

- are endowed with a far superior education than the Hollywood stereotype would lead us believe. They are astute, sophisticated, have an appreciation for consumer psychology, and are receptive to ideas from unusual sources.

In any case, the process of "psychologizing" cigarettes had already begun after World War I when Dr. A.A. Brill, America's first psychoanalyst and translator of Freud's books, began doing work for Lucky Strike during the nineteen twenties. At the outset, he made two points that could be read as the strategy positions for two popular brands on the market today. First, he said that women would interpret cigarettes as a torch of freedom, which is still the sales message behind brands like Philip Morris' Virginia Slims. Then he said cigarettes originally had a male sexual significance which, as we will see, is still the basic appeal of brands like Camel.

Being adept at marketing and willing to peer into the public's psyche is not all that the cigarette companies have done. They have also ventured into the wider arena of public attitudes where their success may have been mixed but still has been innovative. In attempting to deflect the tide of negative public opinion, companies like Philip Morris and RJ Reynolds launched prominent campaigns, but with vastly different results. In the mid-eighties, Reynolds, which has always been the less subtle interpreter of the climate, produced a series of ads that did not push their brands but purported to discuss the "issues." Their campaign claiming that smoking's dangers were merely a matter of scientific controversy that could be easily resolved in a civilized fashion earned them plenty of attention but then backfired; public groups roundly opposed the campaign and the FTC forced them to eat many of their claims and run public retractions.

Philip Morris, which has always had the better appreciation for the profundities of their business, sponsored a series of religious art exhibits. First was The **Vatican Collections: The Papacy and Art** and then the **Precious Legacy** of Jewish art saved from the fires of the holocaust. Later, they found a collection of Episcopalian art to display around the country, and in 1998 Philip Morris of Guatemala even stepped in to restore a defiled Mayan ruin, offering more money than their cigarette sales in that country brought in. A Philip Morris spokesperson explained that the Mayans had introduced the practice of smoking and this was kind of homage.("To Save Mayan Artifacts From Looters, a Form of Protective Custody" **NewYork Times**, Section E, p 31, March 1, 1998) Collectively, however, these efforts have greatly increased the pious legitimacy or what might be called the "spirit power" of Phillip Morris cigarette brands. This is no small issue, because cigarettes are connected to issues of life and death. Cigarette companies are not unaware of this, and even though they are a secular product in this culture, tobacco continues to have a religious function in more primitive cultures. For Reynolds, which attempted to use logic to explain an unnatural practice, the outcome of their campaign has been cataclysmic, eventually showing up in the widespread opposition to their attempt at a new kind of cigarette called Premier and the ostracism of their cartoon spokescamel. For Philip Morris, which seems to have understood the logic of myth and imagination, it has helped the company go on to become one of our largest advertisers and a Fortune 10 corporation of America.

As the tobacco companies try to negotiate their new role as public-bad-guy-cum-major-tax-provider, Philip Morris' seemingly public spirited approach sustains the subtle power that cigarette companies can have on culture: they can reach us through the messages through their current advertising, the ubiquity of their packs in use, and the many cultural events they sponsor. This approach also appears in the marketing strategies they must use to win over the young smokers needed to replace the dying generation and the people who are quitting or cutting back. That, in turn, brings us back to the issue of initiation.

Since smokers tend to be extraordinarily loyal to a particular brand, the tobacco people's claims that advertising is designed only to get smokers to switch is mostly nonsense. Brand advertising not only shapes people's perceptions of the brand they would like to smoke - years before they take to the habit - but it also helps to sell smoking in the first place by creating a sense of inevitability: kids still see it as inevitable to follow in the footsteps of their smoking parents. Most importantly, only cigarettes that have any kind of appeal for youth are advertised, while brands like Pall Mall and Chesterfield, which do not usually appeal to young people, either use very little advertising or none at all. That tends to support the idea that their older smokers, once hooked on the brand, rarely change brands (although they will interchange with knock-off brands to save money) and if teenagers can't be expected to buy a particular brand, why advertise.

It is usually quite easy for cigarette companies to claim they are not trying to reach the young because they don't use teenagers in their ads. But they don't need to use teenagers to reach teenagers because the key is in generating images of an idealized adult lifestyle teens can aspire to. Part of the idea is to show that someone older and presumably wiser *has been there before, so it can't be that bad*. In other words, teenagers understand they are being offered more than just a new kind of habit, they are being offered a path to adulthood. As Marshall Blonsky points out in his conversation with French adman Jacques Séguéla, in **American Mythologies**, "The Marlboro cowboy is fifty years old.....he's completely master of himself. He's passed through the years of desire to the other side. It's security, serenity he signals."

The unfortunate part is that most teenagers who recognize the Marlboro man as the "keeper" of our mythological flame, the symbol who passes on the inner knowledge of the tribe, and then start smoking, will most likely remain smokers. Studies have shown that the earlier in life people start smoking, the longer they are likely to stay with it. People who begin smoking past the age of 21 will find it much easier to quit than people who begin at 16. The result of smokers being stuck with this habit is shown in our national mortality figures: 1 in 6 American fatalities or 400,000 people every year die from smoking-related illnesses.

The problem now is that advertising has done its work. The major brands are so entrenched that tobacco companies do not *need* to advertise the way they did in the past and they can easily live with new restrictions on cigarette advertising. Their ads no longer have to establish the brands; rather, they need only to remind people. Even restrictions on advertising to teens, such as keeping billboards away from schools, are a start, but teens don't only look at ads in the vicinity of schools, they also see them everywhere. Their proximity to schools is just a challenge to the authorities, a cognitive dissonance and an insult to those good folks who believe that society is moral.

But that in itself will not change young minds when it comes to smoking because the ad medium is not the message. The message is that teenagers want to grow up and are searching for a path along with the appropriate symbols and the emotional protection - all the accouterments of adulthood at street level - and they will pick up on that message on any street or magazine they happen to see. Just because the models are adults hardly means that the message is for adults only - teens don't necessarily expect to get their tribal knowledge from other teens.

As this study will show, the actual communication in tobacco advertising is in a coded symbolic language. With a small amount of creativity, cigarette marketers can easily reinvent this language in such a way as to bypass most of the hurdles of a regulated environment. These regulations typically focus on surface issues anyway and whatever understanding they reflect of the symbolic language, this regulated environment is the superficial flotsam of the past. All it takes is for the cigarette advertising industry to borrow from the current visual argot, from the signs of popular culture itself, to create a symbolic language that they and their smokers understand. Like the special frequencies that only animals understand, the tobacco companies and their devotees will recognize each other and their sad but strangely exhilarating marketing pas de deux will continue virtually unaffected.

II Social Changes

From the point of view of **Cigarette Seduction**, the challenge this current generation faces is not just about trying to discourage the young from smoking. It is about finding new ways to address the power that tobacco companies derive from their role of giving teenagers a means of initiation. The fact is that smoking is a relatively new habit in Western culture, which barely existed before the Industrial Revolution. Our real task then, is to bridge the pre-industrial initiation rites that gave teenagers their sense of tribal acceptance with a viable modern solution. One approach, which is an area the cigarette companies long ago targeted, is sports. Unfortunately, although sports gives us a starting point, it remains a partial solution to smoking because it doesn't address many of the intellectual and emotional needs of adolescents: it doesn't apply equally to both sexes, classes, intellectuals, or, for that matter, rebellious types. Nor do sports accommodate the fears and preoccupation that youth has about sex. Cigarettes, on the other hand, have a long association with sex, which is another reason why they are way ahead of sports when it comes to replacing what appears to be our innate need for initiation. To truly resolve the issue of teen smoking we need to provide other approaches to adulthood or we will simply leave a vacuum to be filled by something worse.

Cigarette Seduction is not necessarily an anti-smoking, book since there may well be a place in the cosmos for smoking. Many tribal religions, including contemporary versions of African creeds, such as Santeria, consider smoking a ritual link to altered states. Like most cultural practices that were once tied to religion - art, dance, singing and the consumption of spirits - smoking tends to remain in the modern collective unconscious as an informal but nonetheless mythically charged link to a greater power. No successful tobacco company can be unaware of this and nor, perhaps, should we.

Along with the issue of smoking are the dilemmas of how to adapt as we move from the fading post-Industrial Age to the new realities of the Information Age. When dealing with this kind of change we usually have to look back at our origins to see which practices seem to have become dormant but, nonetheless, are worth reviving. Often these practices will have been carried forward anyway, but in a clandestine, destructive way, and we need to recognize that. Initiation is one of those basic human needs that have been overlooked, and cigarettes have filled that void - but at a price. In this new millennium we will face the growing challenge of reconciling ancient human needs with the new demands of an age inundated with information along with a lingering sense of alienation from nature.

Cigarette Seduction is not about understanding smoking to death, as if that were possible. Decoding cigarettes may be illuminating but that is not the same as destroying smoking. For some people, this decoding could add to its allure. But it does reveal a kind of street semiotic. It tells us about looking at the human message behind the brands. Understanding its argot may help us discover an alternate passage to adulthood that combines the risks of youth and genuine rituals of acceptance with the needs of our increasingly rarefied culture of technology, arts, and knowledge management. We will probably have to look into our primitive selves to find it. If we don't, companies like Philip Morris will continue doing it for us with a commercialized, destructive but highly effective mythology of their own creation.

The first story of smoking then, is about why we start. The next story is why we stay with it and what the brands tell us about the individual who smokes them. The final story is about the language of symbolism: how it communicates our inner needs and how it can be redirected so we no longer need to smoke.

CHAPTER 1: THE MYTHIC SEDUCTION OF SMOKING

It's not that cigarettes are complicated – although there is a lot more to it than you probably thought – it's that you *are complicated. Cigarettes are a blank enough canvas that marketers – and* you *– can bring all the dreams, yearnings and fantasies that you desire to this practice.*

This book takes its cue from one of the great popular enigmas of the late 20th Century: If smoking is deadly, and everyone knows it, then why do 50 million Americans continue to do it? And what about the hundreds of millions more worldwide?

Once upon a time, people thought smoking was a relatively harmless custom, just a habit. During World War I when someone like Henry Ford, in a fit of outrage that seems beyond the call of his duties as head Model T-maker, produced a booklet on smoking called "The Little White Slaver," the public had a good laugh. Back then, smoking was considered to be a raffishly likable habit, a minor human foible perhaps, but probably offset by its value as a social, calming device.

Now that we know otherwise, we look back in amazement at those early ads. In the mid- twentieth century, the tobacco industry competed with outrageous ads that claimed not only was smoking harmless but it was actually recommended by doctors. For example,"More Doctors Smoke Camels Than Any Other Cigarettes," blared one infamous Camel ad in the late nineteen forties.

We may be wiser and more knowledgeable today, but the real lure of the advertising and the imagery remains a mystery to us. Just why *would* people start smoking - and *continue* to smoke - at this time when every veil, every wisp of justification for the habit has been ripped away by overwhelming medical evidence of its trail of destruction. What *is* it about this tobacco that attracts people in spite of themselves?

Regardless of the merits or otherwise of the lawsuits, the truth is that even as they downplayed it, people always suspected that smoking was unhealthy. Some were downright outspoken about it. Meta Lander, in her 1885 book entitled "The Smoking Problem," wrote a chapter devoted to what was then called "smoker's cancer." Since cigars and chewing tobacco were the order of the day, she was referring to mouth and tongue lesions. Others were more concerned about smoking's moral dangers, as if sensing that anyone who would tolerate such self-destruction would also be morally suspect. Lord Baden-Powell, founder of the Boy's Scouting movement, banned smoking among his recruits in 1907 because of its evil influence. In the nineteen twenties, Lucy Gaston, pushing the limits of the prohibition era even tried running for President on the anti-cigarette ticket ("cigarette face" is what she termed the

Republican nominee, Warren Harding), perhaps anticipating one of the themes of the 1996 Clinton-Gore presidential campaign. She, however, lost and died of an unexplained case of throat cancer or being hit by a trolley – depending on whom you believe.

The conclusive, scientifically measurable evidence we have today has turned what was once a real argument between smokers and do-gooders into a modern version of the Flat Earth debate: only a fool would deny that smoking is unhealthy. Yet, even though the proportion of smokers in society has dropped to about 25% today from almost 50% of males in the nineteen forties, their absolute numbers - about 50 million - has been constant for the past 20 years. Many of those smokers are intelligent, functioning beings, people we respect, people like the late Robert Goizuetta, the fabulously successful chairman of Coca-Cola and a chain smoker who died in 1998 of lung cancer.

The reason smoking endures is that it responds to the larger issues of the human dilemma. It eases the way we face the slings and arrows of living. It boosts our sense of self while covering over the rough spots. We don't have to feel as weak, and to the outside world, our weakness is concealed by what is in effect, a smokescreen. The main thing is that once you smoke you really can't just go on in life without it. It is a friend, a confidant and control device, a joy and a source of personal empowerment. There is immense psychological power in the cigarette. It is mysterious to most of us, yet it is always apparent to smokers, especially when they have separated from it. It is the mayonnaise of the psyche, having no particular flavor but bringing all the other flavors to life. It is a kind of sensory lubricant. To the smoker it is a mild, even subtle drug whose specific purpose is defined by the brand and, to a contributory extent, the advertising.

The brand holds the real message and it always tells us about the smoker. Every brand a person has smoked expresses a relationship between them and an effectively marketed message about human yearning. As the smoker chooses a brand, it leaves a kind of audit trail of the smoker: a mirror to the soul that can tell us, once we grasp its essentials, not only why people smoke but something about who they really are when they choose a brand.

Smokers form a relationship with their brands, and the brands smokers choose provide a unique insight into their personality. Just knowing the meaning of popular brands from the way they were developed and then advertised gives us a quick take on the smoker we meet. This could be a distinct advantage in business or in social occasions. It is also the key to unlock the mystery of why people smoke. What is unique about smoking is that it is so subtly mind-altering that the psychology of the smoker is more important than the drug. If we unravel the psychology of why we smoke we may also learn something about the relationships we make with all mind-altering products.

Tobacco was the first valuable product Europeans found in America. Christopher Columbus was first introduced to tobacco by the Indians of San

Salvador in 1492 and was introduced in Spain where it caught on. The 1820 opera Carmen was about a cigarette roller. (Actually, she hand-rolled small cigars called cigarillos). In the seventeenth century Sir Walter Raleigh popularized smoking in England, even running into the opposition of King James. And in courts throughout Europe tobacco was consumed in the form of snuff.

When the British settled in Jamestown it was tobacco-growing that sustained them. There never was a fountain of youth, though some imagined tobacco to be it. There was no El Dorado, no city of gold, except the plantations turning out this very profitable tobacco plant. The new settlers then evangelized tobacco to Europe, growing fat on the profits and the Europeans took it across the world via their spice and silk routes to the East. Then they refined the original tough-to-inhale tobacco, added mass production and developed what has become a deadly breath of life to millions of people around the world.

Any product that can succeed without any apparent benefit, other than it addicts the user, cannot be ordinary or without meaning. Nor is it a practice that will disappear anytime soon. Even as we are seeing tobacco companies actually admit that smoking may indeed be quite dangerous, and adults are obviously quitting in record numbers, there is an increase in cigar smoking. Just when we thought their noxious fumes were a thing of the past, the smell of cigars is back and the ritual goes on in what people hope is not an addictive form of smoking, a kind of revocable cigarette, a "weekenders" smoke.

What magic is there in smoking that keeps people coming? What is it that gets teens to commit and adults to hang on.? What does smoking have so that when one form - cigarettes - becomes declassé, another form - cigars - makes a headline actress like Demi Moore want to appear on the cover of **Cigar Aficionado** smoking one?

To understand what smoking is you have to begin by seeing it as made up of three parts: the physical addiction to nicotine; the hard-to-unravel cycle of psychological dependency that seems to offer smokers an "intensification" of life, self-control and self-punishment, and then the most interesting part of all - the desire to commune with a force larger than oneself.

In order to turn someone into a smoker, there has to be a lure, a compelling, almost magical story that encourages a person to suspend his or her rational faculties and adopt an otherwise unreasonable practice. This is the near mystical element that brings all the parts together and seizes the smoker with an iron grip. After all, if smoking were nothing more than oral reassurance of a primal sort, most intelligent human beings would realize that the health price was too high and the benefit absurd; they would either quit or take to some kind of gum or lozenge instead. But for the most part they don't, and the reason is that for many, smoking is also a pathway to the more gripping human experience of coming into contact with a mythic presence.

In some ways it is the same need that makes us identify with hero stories, romances, and comic books. The difference is that with smoking you don't just identify with the protagonist, but by inhaling smoke you are being given the opportunity to consume, to ingest its spirit of power and romance.

Patriotism is an example of a consumable, empowering myth people find attractive. Significant numbers of people will respond in times of war by risking their safety for little personal gain; in times of peace, the military can still count on volunteers. The rationale for joining the armed forces may have something to do with educational advantages - holding down a job and getting a free education. But the urge to be part of a volunteer army is driven as much by a sense of belonging to a larger movement concerned with the homeland. People, particularly young people, -- need to belong to something much greater than life, something with mythic qualities, regardless of the possibility of drastic consequences. Smoking is way of acquiring that feeling without signing up.

The vast majority of smokers begin in their teen years. RJ Reynolds' own figures (Washington Post, January 15, 1998; p.1, par. 15) show that as many as 89% begin by the age of 18, so that cigarettes have become a universally recognized gateway to adulthood and have long been considered one of its symbols. As we discover more about the key brands like Marlboro and **Winston**, we see how they speak a language that addresses a yearning for rank and enhanced self-image.

The crucial difference between smoking and other forces of mythic empowerment, such as patriotism, religion, or the esthetics of great art is that *they* can only be enjoyed on the occasions when you are there. Smoking, on the other hand, is entirely portable and you can commune with its power on demand. All you need is the seemingly painless commitment to being a smoker. That is why its invitation to addiction can be so attractive: if you are sucked in by its promise of empowerment, you can take it in just about whenever and wherever you want.

To the committed smoker - the addict - the world doesn't seem possible without a smoke and the charge nicotine delivers to the brain. Physiologically, smoking offers the peculiar dual benefits of being either a slight sedative - a calming influence - or a minor stimulant. There is evidence that smokers develop nicotine receptors in the brain that release adrenaline when nicotine reaches it. However, when a lot of nicotine reaches it, such as when smokers are nervous and their breath gets shallower, the act of smoking not only helps deepen the breath but the nicotine clogs the receptors and, by slowing the bodily process, acts as a sedative. Yet smoking would also seem to undermine the breath. So why, we may ask, would something so hazardous to one's health also seem to embolden a person? In moments of stress, tough-guy smokers often do seem to be that much tougher. Lighting that smoke can seem to make one think better, play music more easily, or overcome a blank page or computer screen and write more effectively. It would seem that the loss of breathing power would work against the smoker. Although it *may* do that in the long run, in the moment of need the immediate increase in psychic strength smokers get also explains why they tend to ignore the questions of long-term consequences.

In the nineteen fifties, when the cigarette cancer scare first rocked the country, tobacco companies underwrote the publication of pop psychology articles which served to counteract the health concerns. While recently uncovered evidence has made it clear that tobacco companies used every trick in the book, from manipulating good science to leaning on popular-advertiser supported publications to carry smoker-friendly articles, they also shared something of the truth with the public. The argument they raised was that even if smoking were physically harmful, which the tobacco industry had every reason to doubt in public, smoking was in any case a psychological palliative of sufficient necessity that it more than made up for its health hazards by making people feel better. The most notorious example of this was the **True** magazine special in 1954, which crystallized this point of view in a long article using pseudo-technical language claiming that smokers belong to a personality type with an inherent need to smoke. It even went so far as to say that such people might actually be prone to cancer if they were deprived of cigarettes.

That rationale lingers. Until recently it was on exhibit in the ad pages of such magazines as **Psychology Today,** a quasi-professional journal for mental health specialists which was a highly prized vehicle for cigarette ads. For the smokers themselves, that argument has lived on as their personal rationalization for the habit. There may even be some truth to this because it is generally agreed that there is a psychological component to cancer. So if cancer can have a psychosomatic cause, then it is a short step to believing that dyed-in-the-wool smokers, once deprived of their cigarettes, would be mentally prone to their own form of cancer.

In a peculiar way, Deepak Chopra, the doctor with a sophisticated approach to medicine that combines eastern spiritual enlightenment with western quantum level science, cites a study which may explain why some smokers like Deng Xiaoping can chain smoke into their nineties while others will die early in life with a just a pack-a-day habit. In an experiment by Dr. Herbert Spector of the National Institute of Health, two sets of cats were exposed to cancer drugs and the smell of camphor at the same time. One group of cats was injected with a cancer-killing drug while exposed to the smell of camphor, the others were injected with a cancer-inducing drug that destroys the immune system while exposed to the smell of camphor. Eventually, the cats only had to be exposed to the smell of camphor and their bodies would act as if they had been injected with their respective pro- and anti-cancer drugs. Then both sets of cats were exposed to carcinogens along with the smell of camphor. The cats that had been injected with the anti-cancer drugs were unaffected even though they only had the smell of camphor to protect them. The cats that had learned to associate camphor with cancer-inducing quickly developed tumors and other forms of cancer when they were exposed to the same carcinogens and the smell of camphor. Did the Tobacco Institute have point: that to the properly "programmed" smokers, i.e., those who have an appropriate connection to their brand, a cigarette may work in the same way the camphor did with the cats exposed to its smell and the anti-cancer injections?

Granted, the smell of camphor is not inherently carcinogenic the way smoke is but it does raise some interesting psychosomatic questions: is there some psychic force that pulls us to smoking and why do some survive it while others die young? Whatever the true medical answer may turn out to be, it would be a mistake to look at the practice of smoking through the lens of reasoned argument. Its power and allure clearly belong in another realm of consciousness. Indeed, the best way to understand the psychic appeal of smoking, how it really works, why people want it so badly and why they seem to gather strength from it, is to look at the cult ceremonies, the trance-inducing rituals of pre-Christian religions like those in Southern Asia, Africa, and the Americas. There you will see people gather together in a way that achieves a visible bond with their local deities whose mythological lives are richly described and well understood in their cultures.

The devotees spend several days before the actual ceremonies, slowly working themselves into trances. Carefully observed by cult overseers, volunteers from the community are exhorted by musicians, drummers, and the chants of a sympathetic audience. At some point they will reach a trance level where they are not only oblivious to pain, but actually assume the powers and characteristics of their cult deity.

Depending on which divinity they follow, once they have achieved the proper trance level they undergo a change of state becoming something like a horse god, as in the annual Kuda Lemping trance ceremony of Java, or a sea demon or warlord. As testament to their possession by this spirit they will put blades, pins, hooks and knives into their bodies without feeling any pain. Some will walk on coals. Chinese cults commonly pour boiling oil over themselves without any sign of burning. Margaret Mead's early film records from the nineteen thirties show a ceremony in Bali where people in deep trances engage in ritual battles where they actually stab each other with swords to no apparent ill effect. In the nineteen eighties, the Blair Brothers produced a cultural anthropology travelogue on the tribes and peoples of the islands of South East Asia and showed the same ceremony. The Blairs' footage may be in color and the filming is steady, while Mead's was jerky and in black and white -- but the experience, despite the 50 year gap, was exactly the same: men with otherworldly expressions careen about an open field astride hobbyhorses wielding squat stabbing swords. Once seen, this is not an image easily forgotten. These are adults pushing about what look like Victorian-era toys: horseheads on a pole with a black-and-white checkered saddlecloth. In a peculiar dance of dementia they take great swipes at each other with their swords but none register pain and there is no evidence of cuts or any other injury.

When the ceremonies begin to wind down and the people are brought out of their trances they often collapse in exhaustion and over time may find themselves physically sapped or even damaged from their excursions into altered states. But for the duration of their trances, they have taken on the powers of their idols, which has let them turn pain into a form of strength and perhaps even pleasure. More to the point, they have not just consumed some fetish portion of the spirit power; they have *become* the spirit making *its* power theirs for the duration of the trance.

When we look at smoking we are not looking at a product like soap or candy. This is a product that leads people to believe their spirit is being sustained and their hold on life is being reinforced. Smoking has less to do with the marketplace of ordinary goods than it does with the world of the trance experiences. If you remove the overtly religious aspect and the belief in mythic gods and then replace it with the power of image and advertising in cigarette brands, you could say that we have marketing archetypes – *marketype* - where folk religions have deities. Both are essentially human conceptions that promise unexplainable powers. If you take the trance and reduce its intensity to a momentary sensation of concentrated breath empowerment, and then, if that deep breath were also fueled by a mild nicotine drug and a willing suspense of disbelief that enables otherwise rational people to ignore its dangers, you have the basic appeal of smoking. And further, if you replace the music and chanting with the constant exhortations of the media where the billboard idols have taken on the role of the deities, you will understand why people can feel compelled to smoke, regardless of the long-term effects. Smoking lets people become the god that advertising promises and that our culture demands: if you are an American, you can become the cowboy-knight of Marlboro country or Virginia Slims' lithe, feminist seductress whose puff of independence signals that she has it all. If you are French, you could be the chauvinist with bedroom eyes smoking Gauloise (whose winged helmet conjures up the spirit of the fighting Gauls). Or if you are English you could imagine your place in the Burke's Peerage of your mind because your brand has a royal crest.

Whatever the culture, whatever its demands, tobacco provides the deeply felt illusion that it can deliver what you cannot otherwise have. And it can do it on demand throughout the day.

That is why smoking endures in spite of the health warnings. After all, is not health of the spirit also important? And what price *should* the secular convert pay for it? More to the point - what are the alternatives? As long as it enables people to draw power through their breath, smoking is beyond the range of rational discourse and in the realm of the imagination and the world of personal enhancement. It is this key element which makes smoking so durable and is in effect, a kind of product benefit that the smoker cannot easily forgo, no matter how much he or she matures.

The act of breathing itself is primordial and often part of the mysticism of many religions. Ernest Dichter, founder of motivational or "depth" research in advertising (the use of Freudian analysis of the unconscious in consumer research that helped fuel advertising's post-World War II revolution in marketing) provided a lot of insight on this issue during the nineteen forties.

It was his psychological insight behind such campaigns as the tiger in your tank, the emergence of the shoe as a fashion object ("don't sell shoes," he told his clients, "sell beautiful feet"), the deep meaning of the freezer (a kind of womb), and the convertible as not just a great car but as a stand-in mistress.

If there were one person who could be described as the key influence behind the modern cigarette brand, it is Dichter. Arriving here as an Austrian émigré just one step ahead of the Nazi anschlüss, Dichter inspired a revolution in American marketing. When he left Europe as a renegade, it was both as a potential victim of Nazism but also as a psychoanalytical psychologist who wanted to "sell out the profession" to the lowly world of marketers.

Starting in 1939, he was hired by CBS to analyze the meaning of its soap operas and determine how to keep the story lines relevant to their growing audiences. He soon consulted to such American icons as Proctor & Gamble where he informed his clients that Ivory Soap appealed to a puritan ideal that cleanliness was not only next to godliness but that each shower was also an act of spiritual cleansing and renewal. Soon Ivory's 99 44/100% pure gave way to "Get a Fresh Start With Ivory Soap." That went on to inspire the evangelical urge of soap competitor Dial: "Aren't You Glad You Use Dial. Don't You Wish Everyone Did."

As Dichter racked up successes in this industry it wasn't long before he came to the attention of the cigarette companies. He made sure they noticed him when, in 1947, he published an open letter to the industry, stating that they were "killing themselves" with advertising that touted the supposed benefits of smoking and their "our-brand-is-less-damaging-than-the-other-guys'" approach. This was a product for the psyche, not the body, he proclaimed and the health claims, he predicted, would backfire on the industry.

In 1947, he published a report entitled **Why Do We Smoke Cigarettes** and as he listed the benefits of smoking, almost all of which belong in the realm of acting out and ingesting some form of psychic reassurance, he laid the groundwork for the industry's reinvention of the cigarette in the nineteen fifties, the years when Marlboro, **Winston**, Salem, and then later Virginia Slims, Newport, and the rediscovered Camel emerged.

What Dichter set in motion was the uncovering of the psychological rationale for every product in the marketplace. It showed us that each product has a symbolic value - an iconic life - and the marketers who could manipulate this language of status and desire would reap fortunes. His 1947 classic analysis of the smoking rationale was republished in his 1964 book, **Handbook of Consumer Motivations: The Psychology of the World of Objects**, and recently in several Internet websites. In this handbook, Dichter noted the desire of teenagers to be inducted into adulthood, anticipating what became the burgeoning teen culture of post-WW II affluence. He pointed out that smokers like to watch themselves exhale, not only because they find it creative but because they feel it is like breathing out fire or seeing the transmutation of breath into power.

In the nineteen eighties, the TV baddie, Larry Hagman, who was known for his role as **J.R.** on **Dallas,** noted in his video on **How to Quit Smoking in 7 days**, that as an ex-smoker, one of his reasons for smoking was that he enjoyed watching himself exhale smoke. This theme recurs in ads like a recent series for Camel, where a sultry woman breathes smoke embedded with the image of a camel as though it were signal for a knight of the desert to take her away to paradise. Back in the eighties, a Benson & Hedges ad featured a trumpeter enjoying a smoke with the obvious idea of associating his lung power with the power of inhaled smoke. Then there is the association of trumpeting with smoking.

Dichter, who considered himself as much a cultural anthropologist as an ad researcher, liked reaching into the past in order to explain a market situation in the present and concluded that, to a large extent, smoking is a continuation of the breath cult that was part of many early religions. For example, in the Americas, Indian tribes have often used tobacco in religious ceremonies and in Santeria, the Afro-Cuban religion with Yoruban roots, a cigar, which was sometimes smoked with the burning part in the mouth, is used by men and women at the beginning of a cult event that usually involves trances.

The Judeo-Christian tradition holds that in the beginning there was the "word" which is often interpreted in mystical texts as meaning the breath itself, because there could have been no language at the time. The Greeks had cults that followed the breath. In the orient, the concept of breath as a form of power is a fundamental part of meditation and yoga. The awesome Ki or Qu'i power of the martial arts is related to their control of breath. In Kung Fu or Tai Ch'i the practitioner is able to use meditation and breath control to release a kind of adrenal level of physical power. Ki is often translated as the life force or the vital force.

The basic technique of meditation is the repetition of a mantra like an "aum" sound, which is a ritualization of the sound of the breath and is supposed to have a divine link that leads the subject into a state of higher consciousness.

According to Chopra, each sound achieves a certain pitch which releases energy and the mind, by thinking in certain harmonious ways, can create aminos, a process known as neuropeptides. Kung-fu boxers and karate fighters gain their strength not only from knowing the moves but also from applying their breath control. The advantage of smoking is that it implicitly offers this mastery for about $2.50 a pack ($7 in New York by the middle of the first decade of the twenty first century) by giving you the breath control and adrenal payoff without the isolation or effort of meditation. At the same time, the action of taking in breath, imbibing the nicotine, and then expelling smoke, links the smoker to the spirit power of his or her brand.

In effect, it is the psychic mythology of the brand - its "inner fire" - and not necessarily the advertising that lures people. Advertising is just the wind that helps spread the fire, not the fire itself. In its creation, the ads help spread the fire, even helping to shape the meaning. But once established, the ads are no more important than any other from of spreading the word: through merchandising, point of sale, t-shirt, sports sponsorships, and the basic act of young people imitating the brand choices of their elders.

For that reason, many people in the industry believe that advertising really can't make people smoke. They argue that in Italy during the nineteen seventies, after cigarette advertising had been banned, smoking actually increased. There were special conditions, however; the advertising ban coincided with severe economic troubles and smoking rates often increase with unemployment. In Finland, too, the prohibition of cigarette advertising in no way reduced smoking, especially among teens.

Part of this has to do with the way societies pass on their cultural information. In those cultures where advertising is either not as important or as ubiquitous, word of mouth and peer pressure are the major transmitters of social cues. It is not that different in America, except that brand image advertising starts the chain of events in what is not so much a direct inducement to smoke as it is an attempt to mold the imaginative environment, which in turn leads people to select a particular brand.

To some extent, in an old, relatively homogeneous culture like Italy, where people rely heavily on tradition, word of mouth, and commonly understood symbols for their cultural cues, advertising is not critical to getting the word out. In other respects, since there is less advertising, particularly of the iconic Marlboro kind, it doesn't take much to get the image out there. In the United States it is paid media, which performs the lion's share of this function, and most consistently through advertising and point-of-sale marketing. As a result, in America, the image that a cigarette brand exudes via the media and its packaging, which by now has an established graphic language of its own, is crucial. But in Europe, where individuals do not have quite the need to keep defining themselves as we do, recognizable cultural myths are quickly understood and don't require as much advertising.

In Britain, for example, where the key myths deal with royalty and class, most cigarette packs bear a coat-of-arms with a message declaring that the brand is made by companies such as England's State **Express 555**, that announce, "By Appointment to her Majesty the Queen, Suppliers of Cigarettes." The tobacco companies that can't get a royal seal will often settle for a good imitation of one. Or, like the brand **Players**, they will use old seafaring images that hark back to the days when Britain ruled the waves.

Another approach found in Britain that taps into the past uses an even older idea: smoking as a folk-cure. A once popular working-class brand that used this approach is Woodbine, which is named after a twining shrub and ancient herbal remedy of the countryside. The pack is even decorated with a bough of the plant and it has a colorful history of being handed out free of charge to soldiers in the trenches by Geoffrey Studdert Kennedy, a legendary British World War I padre who came to be known as Woodbine Willy.

In France, the two classic myths exploited by cigarettes are, predictably, chauvinism and a misty, slightly decadent romance. One leading brand produced by the state tobacco monopoly is **Gauloise**. Named for the Gauls, one of the ancient tribes of France, which gave the country its name in Roman times, it is a male brand which, with its chauvinistic title and ancient winged helmet, recalls France's war myths. The other is **Gitanes**, which means gypsy, and is aimed mostly at women, with imagery that is highly evocative of the sensual allure of turn-of-the-century Paris of the Pigalle and Toulouse-Lautrec.

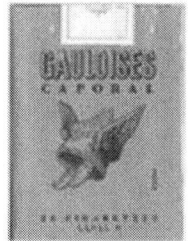

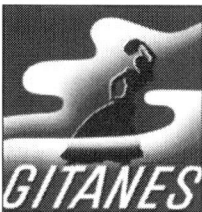

In the end, the reason smoking has survived in the face of all the terrible evidence against it is because it evades human reason by appealing to our desire to be in touch with an iconic power of the culture. Medical authorities may bandy about the concept of addiction and the prevalence of advertising as the reason that people smoke. But people don't become addicted in the first place unless they have a compelling reason to do so. We will see in later chapters that what drives them is a residual need for infantile pacification and self-control combined with a desire to merge with a larger-than-life force. That is why the essence of smoking is not in the advertising but in the brands and in their positioning. Even the tobacco companies recognize this. According to RJ Reynolds' 1984 secret strategic market research documents entitled "Younger Adult smokers: Strategies and Opportunities," by Diane Burrows, released through the discovery process in a lawsuit the company is facing in Minnesota: "The 1983 Segment Description Study showed that *younger smokers are most*

likely to base their brand perceptions on the people they see using the brand -- more than its advertising, package or name." In other words, the brand is the thing and the potency of its message is expressed by the people seen using it. They are its ambassadors and its living billboards and, bar far, its most effective salespeople. The ads exist to add spin and they are constantly changing, with entirely new campaigns being rolled out every three to five years. Yet the packaging of successful brands like Marlboro haven't changed in over fifty years. And when the packaging does change, as in the case of **Winston**, it is usually extremely subtle because there is so much at stake when the appearance is tampered with. The package is the visual expression of the product's "magic," the living link between its generations of smokers and the repository of the brand's DNA.

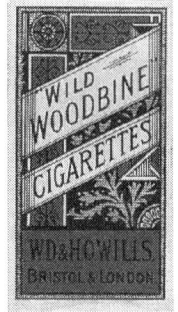

When it comes to understanding what smoking really means to smokers, the place to look is not on the billboards but on the pack where the real message of smoking lies.

Why Do We Smoke Cigarettes?
from *The Psychology of Everyday Living* By Ernest Dichter (1947)

None of the much-flaunted appeals of cigarette advertisers, such as superior taste and mildness, induces us to become smokers or to choose one brand in preference to another. Despite the emphasis put on such qualities by advertisers, they are minor considerations. This is one of the first facts we discovered when we asked several hundred people, from all walks of life, why they liked to smoke cigarettes. Smoking is as much a psychological pleasure, as it is a physiological satisfaction. As one of our respondents explained: "It is not the taste that counts. It's that sense of satisfaction you get from a cigarette that you can't get from anything else."

Smoking is Fun

What is the nature of this psychological pleasure? It can be traced to the universal desire for self-expression. None of us ever completely outgrows his childhood. We are constantly hunting for the carefree enjoyment we knew as children. As we grew older, we had to subordinate our pleasures to work and to the necessity for unceasing effort. Smoking, for many of us, then, became a substitute for our early habit of following the whims of the moment; it becomes a legitimate excuse for interrupting work and snatching a moment of pleasure. "You sometimes get tired of working intensely," said an accountant, whom we interviewed, "and if you sit back for the length of a cigarette, you feel much fresher afterwards. It's a peculiar thing, but I wouldn't think of just sitting back without a cigarette. I guess a cigarette somehow gives me a good excuse."

Smoking is a Reward

Most of us are hungry for rewards. We want to be patted on the back. A cigarette is a reward that we can give ourselves as often as we wish. When we have done anything well, for instance, we can congratulate ourselves with a cigarette, which certifies, in effect, that we have been "good boys." We can promise ourselves: "When I have finished this piece of work, when I have written the last page of my report, I'll deserve a little fun. I'll have a cigarette."

The first and last cigarette of the day are especially significant rewards. The first one, smoked right after breakfast, is a sort of anticipated recompense. The smoker has work to do, and he eases himself into the day's activities as pleasantly as possible. He gives himself a little consolation prize in advance, and at the same time manages to postpone the evil hour when he must begin his hard day's work. The last cigarette of the day is like "closing a door." It is something quite definite. One smoker explained: "I nearly always smoke a cigarette before going to bed. That finishes the day. I usually turn the light out after I have smoked the last cigarette, and then turn over to sleep."

Smoking is often merely a conditioned reflex. Certain situations, such as coming out of the subway, beginning and ending work, voluntary and involuntary interruptions of work, feelings of hunger, and many others regulate the timetable of smoking. Often a smoker may not even want a cigarette particularly, but he will see someone else take one and then he feels that he must have one, too.

While to many people smoking is fun, and a reward in itself, it more often accompanies other pleasures. At meals, a cigarette is somewhat like another course. In general, smoking introduces a holiday spirit into everyday living. It rounds out other forms of enjoyment and makes them one hundred per cent satisfactory.

Smoking is Oral Pleasure

As we have said, to explain the pleasure derived from smoking as taste experience alone is not sufficient. For one thing, such an explanation leaves out the powerful erotic sensitivity of the oral zone. Oral pleasure is just as fundamental as sexuality and hunger. It functions with full strength from earliest childhood. There is a direct connection between thumbsucking and smoking. "In school I always used to chew a pencil or a pen," said a journalist, in reply to our questions. "You should have seen the collection I had. They used to be chewed to bits. Whenever I try to stop smoking for a while, I get something to chew on, either a pipe or a menthol cigarette. You just stick it in your mouth and keep on sucking. And I also chew a lot of gum when I want to cut down on smoking...."

The satisfied expression on a smoker's face when he inhales the smoke is ample proof of his sensuous thrill. Habitual smokers acknowledge the immense power of the yearning for a cigarette, especially after an enforced abstinence. One of our respondents said: "When you don't get a cigarette for a long time and you are kind of on pins, the first drag goes right down to your heels."

The Cigarette -- A Modern Hourglass

Frequently the burning down of a cigarette functions psychologically as a time indicator. A smoker waiting for someone who is late says to himself, "Now I'll smoke one more cigarette, and then I am off." One person explained, "It is much easier to watch a cigarette get smaller and smaller than to keep watching a clock and look at the hands dragging along."

In some countries, the farmers report distances in terms of the number of pipes, as, for example, "It's about three pipes from here to Smithtown."

A cigarette not only measures time, but also seems to make time pass more rapidly. That is why waiting periods almost automatically stimulate the desire to smoke. But a deeper explanation of this function of smoking is based on the fact that smoking is ersatz activity. Impatience is a common feature of our times, but there are many situations which compel us to be patient. When we are in a hurry, and yet have to wait, a cigarette gives us something to do during that trying interval. The experience of wanting to act, but being unable to do so, is very unpleasant and may even, in extreme cases, cause attacks of nervous anxiety. Cigarettes may then have a psychotherapeutic effect. This helps to explain why soldiers, waiting for the signal to attack, sometimes value a cigarette more than food.

"With a Cigarette I Am Not Alone"

Frequently, our respondents remarked that smoking cigarettes is like being with a friend. Said one, "When I lean back and light my cigarette and see the glow in the dark, I am not alone any more...." In one sense, a cigarette seems to be something alive. When it is lighted it appears to be awakened, brought to life. In a French moving picture (Daybreak) the hunted criminal, played by Jean Gabin, holds out as long as he has his cigarettes. He barricades himself against the police and stands siege courageously for some time -- until his last cigarette is gone. Then he gives up.

The companionable character of cigarettes is also reflected in the fact that they help us make friends. In many ways, smoking has the same effect drinking has. It helps to break down social barriers. Two smokers out on a date light up a cigarette as soon as they get into their car. "It's just the right start for an evening," they say. Immediately they feel at ease, for they have found an interest they both share.

We could report many true anecdotes to illustrate how cigarettes bring people together. One such story was related by a middle-aged lady: "A long time ago, on a steamer, there was a boy I was quite eager to meet... but there was no one to introduce us.... The second day out, he was sitting at a table right next to me, and I was puffing away at my cigarette. The ashes on my cigarette were getting longer and longer, and I had no ashtray. Suddenly he jumped up and brought me one. That's how the whole thing started. We are still happily married."

"I Like to Watch the Smoke"

In mythology and religion, smoke is full of meaning. It's floating intangibility and unreal character has made it possible for imaginative man to see therein mystery and magic. Even for us moderns, smoke has a strong fascination. To the cigarette smoker, the clouds he puffs out seem to represent a part of himself. Just as most people like to watch their own breath on cold winter days, so they like to watch cigarette smoke, which similarly makes one's breath visible. This explains the emotional attitudes of many toward smoke. "Smoke is fascinating," said one of the people we interviewed. "I like to watch the smoke. On a rainy day, I sort of lie in a haze in the middle of the room and let my thoughts wander while I smoke and wonder where the smoke goes."

The desire to make things is deep-rooted - and smoke is manufactured by the smoker himself. Smoking provides satisfaction because it is a playful, creative activity. This fact was well stated by one cigarette devotee as follows: "It's a fascinating thing to watch the smoke take shape. The smoke, like clouds, can form different shapes.... You like to sit back and blow rings and then blow another rings through the first ones. You are perfectly relaxed."

"Got a Match?"

Some of the appeals of a lighted cigarette derive from the appeals of fire in general. Fire is the symbol of life, and the idea of fire is surrounded by much superstition. In this connection, it is interesting to note that traces of superstition can be seen in the smoking habits of modern man. For instance some people never will light three cigarettes on one match. It is said that this superstition is based on experiences during World War I. As three soldiers were lighting up the third man was hit when the light of a match flared up for the last time. Our custom of lighting another smoker's cigarette for him may sometimes have an erotic significance, or it may serve as a friendly gesture. Match and cigarette are contact points.

Smoking Memories

Certain moments in our lives are closely linked with cigarettes. These situations often leave on people's memories an important imprint never to be forgotten. Here is such an occasion, described by an office clerk of twenty-one. "...I can remember the moments when I returned home - no matter how late - after having been out with a girl on a Saturday night. Before going to bed, I'd sit on the fire escape for a while and enjoy a smoke. I'd turn around so that I could see all the smoke going up. At the same time, the windows would be bright with lights on the other side of the courtyard. I would watch what the people were doing. I would sit, and watch, and think about what my girl and I had talked about and what a nice time we had had together. Then I'd throw the cigarette away and go to bed. I feel these were really the most contented moments in my life...."

"I remember one time we were in North Africa on a trip and it was evening," said one of our respondents, a nurse about twenty-seven years of age. "During the day, I had noticed there was a lovely spot to sit, across the way from the hotel where we were staying. I went there at night, and sat looking at the stars and the tall cypresses illuminated against the night sky. I was far away in my thoughts. I was thinking of God and the beautiful world he had made. The smoke from my cigarette rose slowly into the sky. I was alone, and at the time I was a part of all the world around me...."

Smoking Mannerisms

Usually the way we smoke is characteristic of our whole personality. The mannerisms of smokers are innumerable. Some people always have cigarettes drooping from their mouths. Others let the cigarette jump up and down in their mouths while they are talking. Men sometimes complain about the way women smoke: "A lot of women blow out the smoke with a gust of wind, right into your face. They just puff it at you." Some men, when they want to appear to be aggressive, hold their cigarettes with thumb and forefinger so that the glowing end shows toward the palm of the hand.

Often smokers will assume a pose, because they have found that it fits their personality best, or at least they think so. A not too modest glamour girl revealed to us some of her "smoking secrets": "I think it looks so much better to smoke with a holder. I studied that very carefully. Don't you think I'm somewhat of a Latin type? It all really depends on what type you are.... I always have holders that are long and dark. I think a long holder is somewhat like a big hat: it's alluring and 'don't dare come close' at the same time."

While every smoker has to go through the motions of lighting and inhaling the smoke, the way in which these acts are carried out varies according to his mood. The nervous smoker has a faster smoking tempo than the relaxed one. The angry smoker blows the smoke in an aggressive way, almost as if he were trying to blow somebody down. A smoker who is about to ask for a raise in salary will press his lips tightly around the cigarette as if to gain courage by holding it that way.

"Smoking Helps Me Think"

The mind can concentrate best when all outside stimuli have been excluded. Smoking literally provides a sort of "smoke screen" that helps to shut out distractions. This explains why many people who were interviewed reported that they couldn't think or write without a cigarette. They argued that moderate smoking might even stimulate mental alertness. It gives us a focal point for our attention. It also gives our hands something to do; otherwise they might make us self-conscious and interfere with mental activity. On the other hand, our respondents admit that smoking too much may reduce their efficiency.

Cigarettes Help Us to Relax

One shortcoming of our modern culture is the universal lack of adequate relaxation. Many of us not only do not know how to relax, but do not take time to learn. Smoking helps us to relax because, like music, it is rhythmic. Smoking gives us a legitimate excuse to linger a little longer after meals, to stop work for a few minutes, to sit at home without doing anything that requires effort. Here is a nostalgic comment contributed by a strong defender of smoking: "After a long day's work, to get home and sit in a chair and stretch my legs 'way out, and then to sit back and just smoke a cigarette and think of nothing, just blow the smoke in the air - that's what I like to do when I've had a pretty tough day." The restful effect of moderate smoking explains why people working under great stress use more tobacco.

"I Blow My Troubles Away"

In times of high tension, cigarettes provide relief, as indicated by the following typical comments of one of our respondents: "When I have a problem, and it comes back and back, warningly saying, 'Well, what are you going to do about this?' a cigarette almost acts like a consolation. Somehow it relieves the pressure on my chest. The feeling of relief is almost like what you feel in your chest after you have cried because something has hurt you very much. Relaxing is not the right kind of word for that feeling. It is like having been in a stuffy room for a long time and at last getting out for a deep breath of air." That man's explanation comes very close to stating the scientific reason why smoking brings relief. Worry and anxiety depress us not only psychologically but also physiologically. When a person feels depressed, the rhythm of his breathing becomes upset. A short and shallow breath creates a heavy feeling in the chest. Smoking may relieve mental depression by forcing a rhythmic expansion of the breast and thus restoring the normal pace of breathing. The "weight on the chest" is removed.

This connection between smoking and respiration accounts for the common expression, "Smoking helps us to let off steam." When we are enraged, we breathe heavily. Smoking makes us breathe more steadily, and thus calms us down.

Cigarette Taste Has to Be Acquired

Most people like the smell of tobacco but dislike the taste of a cigarette. Frequently we were reminded that "a cigarette never tastes as good as it smells." One usually very much dislikes his first cigarette. Taste for cigarettes must be acquired slowly. And whenever a smoker tries out a new brand, with a lightly different taste, he finds that he has to repeat this process of becoming accustomed to the taste. Often smokers who say they do not like the taste of certain brands really mean that they are not accustomed to it. Few advertisers of cigarettes realize that it takes time for a smoker to change his taste habits. No matter how pleasant the taste qualities of a brand may seem to be, at first the unaccustomed taste will be disliked. One of our respondents made the following interesting comment on this point: "I went to Bulgaria once and was forced to smoke Bulgarian cigarettes. I tried one brand after another till I had gone through five brands. Finally, the sixth brand seemed to be perfect. I discovered much later that any of the other brands might have become my preferred brand if only I had tried it in the sixth place. It just took me that long to learn to appreciate Bulgarian tobacco."

How Many a Day?

Despite all the millions spent on comparing the potentially harmful effects of different brands of cigarettes, our respondents seemed very little concerned about this matter. But all of them, even those who do not smoke excessively, worry about the quantities they smoke. Scientific and medical studies on the physiological effects of smoking provide a confused picture: Some conclude that smoking is harmful; others deny it. This same confusion prevails among smokers themselves. Nevertheless, all of them worry about smoking too many cigarettes, as shown by the fact that nearly everyone has tried, at one time or another, to "cut down on" smoking. "I'll tell you something I do," one smoker confided. "I give up smoking cigarettes every year for one month, and I say to myself that I'll prove to myself I can still do without them." Periodic abstemiousness of this kind indicates an underlying feeling of guilt. Such individuals really think that constant smoking is not only harmful, but also a bit immoral. Efforts to reduce the amount of smoking signify a willingness to sacrifice pleasure in order to assuage their feeling of guilt.

The mind has a powerful influence on the body, and may produce symptoms of physical illness. Guilt feelings may cause harmful physical effects not at all caused by the cigarettes used, which may be extremely mild. Such guilt feelings alone may be the real cause of the injurious consequences.

The First Cigarette

Much of this guilt feeling can be traced directly to one's first cigarette, which the older generation remembers as a forbidden and sinful thing. Their fathers considered the habit an educational problem, whereas many parents nowadays have adopted a "modern" attitude toward smoking. Here is what one such father said: "I told my son I thought he was a little young... He is seventeen. It might not do him any harm to wait another year or two. Then I remembered my own first cigarette and what awful stuff I had to smoke in secret. In a way, my son is lucky to be able to start with a good cigarette without running the danger of ruining his health. I gave him a pack of the brand I smoke."

Most of us remember vividly the first cigarette we smoked. "I certainly remember my first cigarette," said one of our respondents. "We were a bunch of boys on our way to a football game. I had trouble lighting my cigarette, and at that moment a man passed by and yelled at me: 'Throw that cigarette away, you rascal!' I was so shocked and frightened that I obeyed his command without hesitation. But only a few minutes later, I lighted another one just to demonstrate to myself that I was not afraid.

"No, Thanks, I'll Smoke My Own"

This is the reply of most smokers when they are offered a brand different from their own. Brand loyalty among smokers is strong and persistent. Individuals smoke one brand consistently, so that they become identified with it. A guest who discovers that his host smokes the same brand considers this a personal flattery. If a young lady changes to the brand of an admirer, he understands that he has surely made an impression. Here is the experience of one young man and his interpretation of it: "I was very fond of a girl. She was giving a farewell party before leaving the country. I didn't have any idea how I stood in her affection. The only clue was that at her party she had my brand of cigarettes. I always felt that that was in deference to me." "My brand" has a special significance, as if it were a part of the smoker's credo and personality.

A Package of Pleasure

A new pack of cigarettes gives one a pleasant feeling. A full, firm pack in the hand signifies that one is provided for, and gives satisfaction, whereas an almost empty pack creates a feeling of want and gives a decidedly unpleasant impression. The empty pack gives us a feeling of real frustration and deprivation.

During the seventeenth century, religious leaders and statesmen in many countries condemned the use of tobacco. Smokers were excommunicated by the Church and some of them were actually condemned to death and executed. But the habit of smoking spread rapidly all over the world. The psychological pleasures derived proved much more powerful than religious, moral, and legal persuasions. As in the case of the prohibition experiment in the United States, repressive measures seem to have aroused a spirit of popular rebellion and helped to increase the use of tobacco.

If we consider all the pleasure and advantages provided, in a most democratic and international fashion, by this little white paper roll, we shall understand why it is difficult to destroy its power by means of warnings, threats, or preachings. This pleasure miracle has so much to offer that we can safely predict the cigarette is here to stay. Our psychological analysis is not intended as a eulogy of the habit of smoking, but rather as an objective report on why people smoke cigarettes. Perhaps this will seem more convincing if we reveal a personal secret: We ourselves do not smoke at all. We may be missing a great deal.

CHAPTER 2:
CAMEL -- HOW THE MYTH WAS FIRST BROUGHT TO MARKET

Oddly enough, it took cigarette executives around forty years of experience in mass marketing to identify the quintessential American smoking myth even though they had long understood the potential of symbols in packaging and advertising. In the early days, the selection of a brand image had been strictly a matter of serendipity. Lucky Strike took its name from a brand of chewing tobacco that had been popular with miners. Its name and the bull's-eye logo make the promise literally of consuming a shot of good luck or simply, divine providence, an indication that a smoker's life goals are associated with risk or pure chance. Nowadays, the brand has become associated with the stereotype of a working-class smoker with a retro, fifties view of the world and a willingness to put him or herself at great risk for some unlikely payoff. In 1996 the brand was restaged with tepid success as an "American Original."

Fortunately, even in those early days, the creation of new brands of cigarettes was often documented and it is clear that their successes were a matter of informed taste as well as good luck on the part of the cigarette company executives. Back then, when a tobacco company would decide it needed a new kind of brand, someone would select a packaging idea they liked and, with good luck, it worked. When it came to **Camel** - the first brand with an image expressly created in response to market conditions - it was part planning and part good fortune that in 1913, R.C. Haberkern at Reynolds hit on the idea of using Old Joe, the circus dromedary, as a model for the pack. Named **Camel**, in honor of the two-humped desert animal, the brand settled for the now familiar, one-humped dromedary seen on the pack. A slight twist in the execution of the idea had made all the difference.

At the time, RJ Reynolds just needed to respond to competitive pressures from cigarette brands using Turkish tobacco and a mid-eastern image. Back then, they were competing with **Murad**, the leading brand made from imported Turkish tobacco. Local cigarette companies realized they could compete against them if they blended Turkish tobacco with a coarser domestic variety that had been processed and treated with additives and flavorings that suggested a mid-eastern flavor. The treatment consisted of bleaching white burley tobacco and flavoring it with sugar and chemical "fixings." The cheaper smoke they ultimately produced was a mixture of this; a finer local tobacco called Carolina bright and a dash of the Turkish variety. In tests, this seemed to taste to the American smoker as good as the real thing. The only task remaining was to develop an image

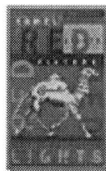

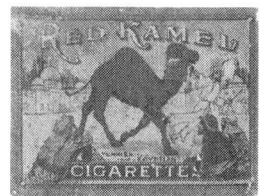

that was both mid-eastern and American.

Once it was decided to call the brand **Camel**, thereby suggesting Turkish quality without making the brand too noticeably foreign, it was just a matter of getting one of their employees to find a model for the pack. Curiously, the packaging was based on a predecessor in Reynolds' stable of brands called **Red Kamel** - which has now been revived using bizarre Generation-X style typography - that also featured a one-humped dromedary. The earlier package showed the beast running, which was appropriate since the dromedary is a racing camel and was bred for speed. Fortunately for Haberkern, Barnum & Bailey's circus happened to be in town when he got his assignment and "Old Joe" their famous dromedary happened to be the closest thing around to the Arabian beast. So he used it as his model and the tradition of having a dromedary instead of a camel was maintained.

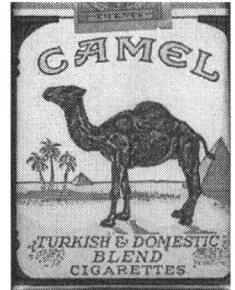

According to Chris Mullen, in his book, **Cigarette Pack Art**, the legend is that "Old Joe" would not remain still for the photographer and his trainer, a tough old fellow in his own right, "whacked him on the nose with a stick. Outraged, 'Old Joe' pulled back his ears, raised his tail and adopted a posture halfway between offended dignity and aggression." The pose has been immortalized by the **Camel** pack and the rest, as they say, is history.

That, at least, is the official story. But it is likely that they had a hunch about the animal's deeper significance. Reynolds had **Red Kamel** on the market for a number of years and although it was not very successful they seemed to have a gut feeling that something about it appeared to make sense. That is why they hung on to the concept. The key was in getting rid of the color red and the Germanic reference (camel with a "K"), and instead of having the camel gallop, they let it stand still and assume a certain look of hauteur. They also seemed to know they needed to stick with the one-humped camel, the dromedary.

When the product was launched in 1914, RJ Reynolds' advertising agency, N.W. Ayer, spent a then fabulous sum of around $700,000 on promoting it. Using what was at that time an innovative technique to win the public's attention - a carefully staged series of teaser ads proclaiming that something new was on its way - the brand became a top seller. One ad went: "Camels! Tomorrow there will be more Camels in this town than in all Asia and Africa combined!" By the nineteen thirties, the famous slogan "I'd Walk A Mile For A Camel" - in other words, humorously reversing the-beast-of-

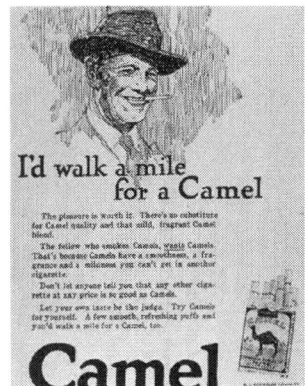

burden metaphor and making the human, in a manner of speaking, the pack animal - entered our lexicon of famous phrases, turning the brand into an icon.

The role reversal is more than a lucky turn of phrase by a copywriter; it was also an unintended reference to addiction: a smoker who finds himself out of cigarettes will gladly walk a mile for his brand. Generally, great cigarette campaigns as well the brand messages themselves have had a double meaning suggesting pain or sufferance in return for pleasure.

A modern reading of the Camel pack has given us a much different view of this beast whose symbolic image transcends its superficial circus and Araby context. Nowadays, especially after the Joe Camel cartoons, it is clear that the camel relates to animal life the same way Georgia O'Keefe's flowers relate to flora. Where O'Keefe's flowers were symbols of female genitalia, it is easy to see nowadays that the dromedary is not just an exotic beast of burden but with its shape - the hump, its long neck and the abundance of hair - it was always the symbol of a penis.

It is little wonder that after old Joe Camel turned into a cartoon with phallic features, it became the lightning rod of protest against the teen tobacco advertising. Yet it took around 10 years before the pressure groups could force a very knowing marketing department at RJ Reynolds to retire the camel they had transformed into an anthropomorph labeled "Smooth Character." For one of the first times in memory, symbolspeak became a matter of public contention as health groups opposed this cartoon on the grounds that it was recognized by kindergartners and that it made sly references to the male genitalia.

Naturally, RJ Reynolds and their ad agency, Mezzina Brown, disavowed any knowledge of the phallic references, just as they have denied it attracted kids. Even the artist who conceived it said it was "a lark." But that hardly matters. If the public perceives it as a kind of penis, then so it is.

The interesting thing about **Camel** is that RJ Reynolds itself had a poor understanding of its symbolic resonance in the early nineteen seventies when they changed the package in the hopes of winning over a newer, more modern smoker. They attempted this by abandoning the desert-and-pyramids background and focusing on the camel only. However, they produced a clinical rendition of a camel, making it significantly less hairy, and took out the background coloring so that the rest of the pack was pure white.

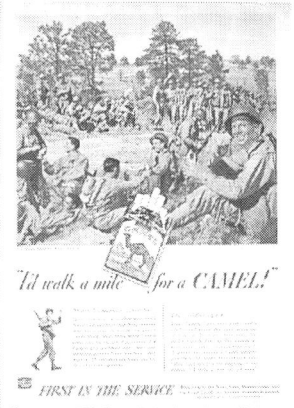

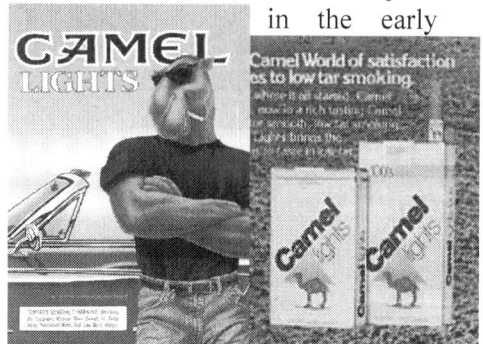

The net effect was a very cold package and a decidedly smooth-looking camel.

The result of abandoning the steamy phallic symbolism of yore was a slump in sales. Before long, the Reynolds people began looking at the old pack with fresh eyes and within a few years the old camel-and-pyramids images were reinstated. Some minor changes were incorporated and sales began to climb again. Apparently, the company had a more intuitive knowledge of human nature in the old days than in the **seventies** decades of expensive consumer research. But with the return to basics, **Camel** once again became a contender. When it got the cartoon it became a top-selling brand in the youth marketplace.

The real question is whether or not people had always made the connection - the unconscious recognition of its phallic message - even though its strongest resemblance to the male parts was perceptible when viewed upside down? There is plenty of reason to believe; according to research in Professor Norman F. Dixon's **Preconscious Processing** (Wiley, 1972), it hardly makes any difference. In matters of food, sex and survival - drive related stimuli - these images belong in a powerful class of their own. These images are recognized at subliminal thresholds and they are as readily understood upside down as right side up, if they make the right suggestion. At a subconscious level, awareness occurs in a way that directly addresses the viewers' imagination and they can be conditioned by advertising stimuli. In a key experiment by two psychological researchers (Silverman & Silverman, 1964, '*A clinical-experimental approach to the study of subliminal stimulation*' Journal of Abnormal Psychology 87, 341-57) they found that exposing a male audience to pictures of a nude female flashed subliminally on a screen using a tachistoscope influenced the way they perceived Rorschach blots afterwards. Likewise, sexy ads and phallic-looking cartoon camels easily reinforce whatever tendency there is for people to view **Camel** as a penis symbol.

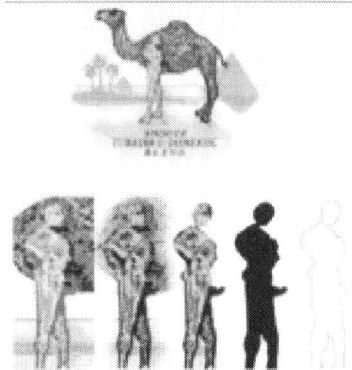

In a research study done in Mexico City schools, a majority of teens identified an engorged male in the legs of the Camel image on a pack. This research was conducted by the Department of Research in Tobacco Smoking of the National Institute of Respiratory Disease in Mexico City from1998 to 1999. with 1,186 adolescents ranging from 12 to 16 years of age.

Since all along, the message of **Camel** has been a plainly phallic one, it tells us something important about the smoker, because the unconscious choices people make are nothing if not honest. Finding the right interpretation can be tricky, though, and making sense of why a smoker has chosen a brand often requires taking into account the unguarded first impression the smoker gives when he or she lights up and faces the world. That is the first opportunity to identify the relationship smokers are making with the brand. Then, by looking at a few other clues, such as the filter type, pack type, length, smoking style, how the cigarette is lit, the way the cigarette is disposed of and, if possible, how the pack itself is discarded, one can put the pieces together. Interpretation is a manageable art that can yield fascinating results by taking into account the obvious details that accompany each brand.

For a deeper analysis, it helps to know the smokers' brand history, what they started with, what they changed to, and so on. Brand changes often coincide with a change in personal circumstances, particularly when **smokers** migrate from their long-term brand choice. When **smokers** change brands a lot, it usually reflects an unsettled period in their life and the brand choices often give a clue to the forces they were contending with. Later chapters will show how to make sense of some of the clues given by brand changes. But before we get there we will take a closer look at the great riddle of why people really want to smoke.

CHAPTER 3:
THE SIREN CALL – A SENSE OF PERSONAL CONTROL

Smoking is now officially recognized as an addiction. As anyone who has come into contact with addiction knows, people who usually "wander" into addiction do so with eyes more open than they would like to admit. The sheer numbers of smokers who readily adopt the practice of smoking despite the face of overwhelming evidence of its hazards strongly suggests they know what they're getting into. It is true that the legality of the product and the ubiquity of its advertising has a way of implying that it can't be that bad. But smokers still know they are getting addicted and the ugly endgame of the product is no secret

One clue to smokers' motivation is what happens when they are threatened with the loss of their cigarettes. They become aggressive and childlike whenever people attack their habit. If you threaten to take it away, they will cling to their drug the way a child hangs on to a rattle. Turning childlike may even be the key, because much of addiction is about recapturing the bliss and dependence of infancy,- but in what the smoker thinks is going to be his or her own terms.

According to medical research, it takes about three days for all trace of nicotine to leave the body. While people like the Surgeon General have said cigarettes are addicting and as hard to quit as heroin, the fact is, if you stop smoking for three days, you have no physical need for nicotine. So if chemical dependency were all, you should no longer need to smoke after those three critical days.

However, as anyone who has tried knows, it is much harder to quit than just having to forgo cigarettes for three days. Most smoke-stop organizations agree that six months after quitting, many ex-smokers hit a critical point where they are highly disposed to resume smoking. What has come back to haunt them after six months is the mental pull of dependence, self-control, and the mythos of the cigarette's imagery.

It may seem hard to reconcile a macho brand like **Marlboro** or **Camel** with the idea of childlike dependence, but it is important to realize that underneath it all the smokers are recreating that dependence in their own terms. It is easy to see that smoking is not only distinctly oral but that also helps explain why the cigarettes themselves, in their most popular form, have an oddly colored "cork-tip" filter. The continued existence of this speckled brown-colored filter has never been explained; it seems to exist without rationale and remains the norm among male-oriented brands. The white-colored tip on the other hand, is the norm among women's brands. All macho filter cigarettes today, such as Marlboro, **Winston**, Kool, and Camel, have cork-colored tips while the leading women's brands, such as Virginia Slims and **Salem**, are white-colored, non-cork tips. It would seem that all cigarettes should have a white tip because it matches the natural color of the cigarette paper. Since that is not the case, the prevalence of the cork-colored tip for men suggests that some mysterious reasoning is at play.

Like most mythic phenomena, the existence of the cork tip has its origins in a situation that has long since lost its relevance. Yet the practice continues for seemingly unfathomable reasons so that its true rationale probably has little to do with its history.

In the early years of the century, when there were no filters, smokers often found that bits of tobacco fell out of the cigarettes and stuck to their lips. One common solution was to tap the cigarette on the pack before lighting it in order to pack the tobacco more tightly into the paper tube. This is a practice you can still see in old black-and-white movies and you can probably recall a few Bogart scenes where he taps a cigarette before delivering one of his trademark lines.

This trick never worked perfectly though, and at that time, back in the twenties, concerned tobacco companies included a small cork cigarette holder with each pack. The smoker kept this holder and used it on all the cigarettes in the pack after which he threw it away. Sophisticated smokers avoided these and bought their own, fancier holders. FDR is remembered today for his extravagant cigarette holders. In their time, cigarette holders evolved into status symbols even though they were generally considered feminine. However, in refined circles men adopted them too, along with a slightly challenging, supercilious attitude along with it. By the nineteen thirties, most smokers had decided that the cork holders were just too clumsy and they lost popularity.

When manufacturing technology did a better job of tamping down the tobacco, and some brands added "mouthpieces" or cardboard smoking tips, the cigarette companies discontinued the cork holders. But the public developed a liking for the cork color anyway and tobacco companies continued offering a cork-colored tip on their cigarettes even though there was no filter, holder, or other device to justify its existence. So the cork color remained at the smoking end of the cigarette for no apparent reason other than that the public seemed to like it. The question is: why is it still there? Products don't usually carry vestiges of previous features unless there is some compelling psychological reason to do so. Usually, as in this case, it transcends its original purpose. For example, when research showed that fire engine red was actually hard for drivers to see, fire engines were quickly recast in Day-Glo green. But many fire companies found that although the engines were more visible, drivers didn't recognize them as fire trucks. As a result, many fire companies incorporated an orange or red color strip on the fire trucks to maintain a connection to the traditional fire engine color.

Clearly, the cork-colored tip stood for something that mostly male smokers were reluctant to give up. A more intriguing question is: why it is that the "he-men," like the Marlboro and **Winston** smokers, want cork colored tips? "....Holding a cigarette in your mouth," said the Madison Avenue motivational researcher Ernest Dichter, after having done basic research into smoking for the J. Stirling Getchell agency back in the nineteen forties, "is comparable to sucking at the nipples of a gigantic world breast and deriving from it the same type of satisfaction and tranquilizing effect that the baby does when being nursed."

The cork-tip in other words, is a substitute nipple. The cork coloring is reminiscent of a nipple and it survived because smoking is largely about oral gratification. At some level you might speculate that the "he-men" smokers just want their mommies. On the other hand, men are supposed to like breasts. In many ways, the smokers drives can be identified with the way they smoke: some take in well-managed puffs, others drag on it as if life itself were about to take leave.

Since we have an established norm - that men generally smoke cork-colored filters and women tend to go with plain white-colored filters - it is possible to make some inferences about individual smokers on the basis of their filter choices, especially when they deviate from the norm. White represents the color of a brassiere or literally, its concealment, whereas men wish for just the opposite. There are limitations, of course. Generally, people choose the cigarette by its brand and the filter just happens to come with it - whatever its color.

A smoker will not stay with a brand if the filter type is inconsistent with the meaning he or she finds in the brand. At the very least, the smoker would experience ambivalence over smoking it, It is not uncommon for people to have misgivings about their favorite brand, in which case they will have one or two alternative brands. However, whenever there is a contradiction of some kind between the smoker's personality and the brand symbolism - for instance, an effete male using a "he man" cork tipped brand - then pure compensation is likely to be at play. These smokers might just as well be announcing that, whatever they lack in their psyche is measurable by the deviation from the brand or cigarette type they *should* be smoking.

One way of looking at this is that the cigarette-dependent macho male has a strong preference for cork-colored filters because he is really an overgrown boy who still needs the comfort of his mother's breast. Women, for the most part, appear to be weaned earlier or, for gender reasons are discouraged from taking too much comfort from the breast. So when you find exceptions to the rule, such as a man smoking a white

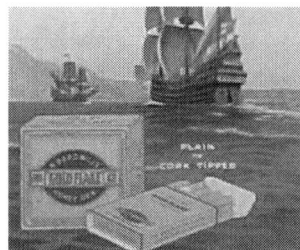

filtered brand like **Kent** or the U.S. version of Benson & Hedges, he may not necessarily be effeminate or better weaned, but, rather he is likely to be somewhere on a continuum from exceptionally discreet to downright deceitful. On the other side of the coin, a woman smoking cork-colored tips is likely to be more open, outgoing, or tomboyish than most, or perhaps even someone like a blues singer with a penchant for men

Filter colors are by far the broadest category of meaning, so there are many exceptions. For example, one would expect a woman who smoked a macho brand to exhibit some degree of assertiveness, even if it were only the submerged, wishful kind. But if she showed no evidence of aggression and the brand was unrealistically masculine, then you suspect that she was finding, in her brand, a substitute for the male she was missing in her life. She may also be more wanton - the "exposed" filter merely signaling that she is available.

Smokers are legendary for their brand loyalty and the deep relationships they form with their cigarettes has its roots in their early oral experiences. Often, it is hard to reconcile the seemingly tough exterior of a smoker with the fact that deep down he or she is responding to their need for a pacifier. What is really taking place is that once smokers have satisfied their need for oral indulgence they are then also empowered to act out their would-be own macho dispositions.

Orality in smoking is a widely accepted concept because it is easy to see the connection between smoking and maternal comfort. But that is just the visible connection between smoking and its origins in childhood. It can go deeper still because smoking also has a relationship to the womb.

One sight that must bring joy to the heart of a tobacco executive is the picture of a developing fetus, because it will show the unborn baby with a thumb near its mouth. The message is that we begin life with the need for oral reassurance and that is the bedrock of this business. The baby, once born, is obviously ready for breast-feeding but there is still a residual relationship with the umbilical cord itself. Breast-feeding and any ensuing orality can also be associated with the original cord of life, which is why any act of imbibing can have deep emotional and spiritual values. It is understandable then, why tobacco ads occasionally try to exploit this impulse, the most significant being a series in the nineteen eighties for Vantage, a now fading RJ Reynolds brand, where men and women were shown in commanding situations, yet somehow being attached to a rope or a length of cable or, in this ad, a glass of adult sustenance - red wine.

Vantage is not an ordinary brand to begin with; it has a unique filter that combines the cork-colored "breast substitute" with a hollow white interior that is suggestive of a belly button or an umbilical cord. Superficially,

Vantage ads have played on their name by putting their smokers in situations where they can look down from a strategic, "vantage" point. But a closer examination of their ad campaigns in the eighties showed that the people were either holding up ropes or being attached to some kind of cabling. Their classic ad showed a diver holding up what looks like a diver's lifeline; in another ad, a sports announcer is shown with headphones that are connected by cable to the "mother station."

At first glance, most of these references appear so incidental as to lack any special significance. But in reality, ads are heavily researched before they are put into publication because there is just too much money spent it for them to be mere accidents. With that in mind, it is hard to look at a Vantage smoker without inferring an unresolved condition based on maternal closeness or some form of self-absorption. When meeting a Vantage smokers, there is a good chance they will be among the unsung philosophers of our times, the local savant to whom no benefit has accrued from their insight, or at some elemental level, they are the kind of people who take pleasure, quite literally, in examining their navels.

The oral rationale for smoking has been demonstrated in psychological experiments, such as Spence & Gordon's 1967 study ("Activation and measurement of an early moral fantasy," Journal of the American Psychoanalytic Association 15, 99-129) showing that when people are subjected to the stress of rejection or unpopularity their desire for oral relief - that is, to suck on something - increases dramatically. Moreover, this can be enhanced by subliminal stimuli. While that helps explain the connection with early childhood and even pre-birth itself, it only tells us about the pacifying quality of smoking. Smoking is more than just a way of dealing with stress because, vexatious as it is, stress can be managed with any number of relaxation techniques, ranging from deep breathing to meditation and visualization.

The fact is that people also smoke when they are not subjected to any stress at all. Many people enjoy smoking during moments of perfect leisure. Smoking in the bathroom is so popular that many smokers consider it an essential part of their toilet activity, thereby adding a level of sensuality to ordinary bodily activities. This is the part of smoking - enhancing ordinary or even pleasurable moments - that takes us beyond the infant dependency side of the habit and gives us the first clues about the darker side of smoking. We know that the nicotine and the oral experience help in recapturing that idyllic stage of early life. We know that people are always susceptible to being drawn back to that time of total protection during pre-birth when they were safe in the womb. It is easy to appreciate the lure of re-experiencing moments of infancy and the extended womb of the nursery with its daily ceremonies of loving care. But how do we go from there to deal with the destructive side of smoking?

The health warnings on cigarettes today are so severe that it is hard to believe any rational person would continue smoking. Who in their right mind would consume something that warns of causing emphysema, cancer and defects to the unborn? In countries like Canada cigarette packs even include graphic warnings with blackened lungs and drooping cigarettes occupying up to 50% of the pack.

According to some anti-smoking authorities like smokEnders founder, Jacquelyn Rogers, there is reason to believe that the health warning may even be a sales inducement. The argument is that, from the point of view of the makers of low-tar brands, the health warning is a useful way of reminding smokers that the brand isn't too weak to be worth smoking.

The addiction factor alone doesn't really explain why 50 million people are willing to ignore the warnings and continue to smoke. Obviously, there is something much deeper taking place in the face of which, the health danger of cigarettes seems minor by comparison. Indeed, so extreme is the price of smoking, that ascribing it to something related to infancy does not go far enough. You have to consider what it is in infancy that makes smoking so compelling. Since the danger theme itself that shows up in smoking is also part of its allure, we can assume that it is related to the love-and-punishment routine that is used by parents and society to raise children. As blissful as those early years may have been, they were also filled with terrors stemming from parents' discipline and the traumas of being weaned and housebroken. The result is that with smoking, the element of danger works in the mind as a vicarious parent, where the prospect of self-injury has taken the place of a parent's chastisement as a means of self-control.

The pleasure-control syndrome is a fundamental element in smoking and it is one that needs to be considered when quitting or sending out quit-smoking messages. It just isn't good enough to say to a smoker, "You will be a better person if you quit." This approach is usually what makes public service ads and personal entreaties to smokers fail. There also have to be suggestions about what smokers can do with their negative feelings, particularly the ones that can work against them. Otherwise, the message will not only fail but will be perceived by the smoker as being insufferably self-righteous.

While not all of us have to plead with loved ones to stop smoking and even fewer of us will be writing anti-smoking commercials, the act of smoking has grown so unreasonable in the light of all we know that it can only be a doorway to another level of the human condition. Because of that, we need an answer, a rebuttal, a way of accommodating tolerance for it. Even the casual observer wonders why someone they meet smokes. In business or social life, they will feel inclined to get a handle on why that person smokes: what *is* it saying about them? Do I *want* to deal with this person or does their smoking signify some mark of negativity that tells me I should avoid them?

To smoke today, is to be judged. That is one of the reasons people have been rushing to cigars, where they can assume a haughty demeanor and use, what is to the spectator, cigars' vile smell and the high cost of the tobacco to defy others' best judgment. But once they pick up a cigarette again, their flaws are merely ordinary and you can judge them. Cigars are no less amenable to symbolic analysis but the cigar revival is still young and the new generation of smokers has yet to develop the kinds of long-term relationships they have with cigarettes. Nor are the brands and the cigar types well enough understood in public consciousness **so** that they have developed the level of meaning we can draw from highly advertised and much used cigarette brands.

On the other hand, the dynamics are roughly similar: behind every smoker is a positive-negative polarity that governs the relationship they make with their brand. With cigar smokers the brand is often a matter of region: Cubans at the top, and Dominicans just below with brands like Monte Cristo, and then Mexicans with TeAmo and machine-made stogies with inferior tobacco at the bottom. We can understand why, as with cigarette smokers, weak people often smoke strong brands and strong people sometimes smoke bizarre brands. The difference is that strength, weakness, and in case of cigars "good taste," is expressed in the shape of the cigar as well as the presumed quality of the tobacco. Generally, cigar smokers choose the shape according to their own body size and their own sense of status. That is why a diffident man might smoke a panatela while a captain of industry, if he thought of himself as a fat cat, would go for a Churchill. In either case there is meaning in their choices and it is the variety of combinations that make the art of interpretation so interesting.

CHAPTER 4:

"CRACK" vs. LEAF – ORIGIN OF THE CIGARETTE

Before getting into the personality of modern brands and the evolution of their meaning, it is worth taking a look at the prehistory of cigarettes - the world back when there were no brands and tobacco was essentially a commodity. Cigarettes themselves are a recent development. They are supposed to have originated in the nineteenth century, when a new "kind" of tobacco called Bright was inadvertently produced in 1839 by a slave. By applying sudden heat to the curing of an otherwise cheap, inferior variety of burley tobacco, he produced a yellowish, mellow-tasting substance that could be inhaled when smoked. Traditional forms of tobacco, the kinds Columbus found the Indians smoking when he first arrived in the Americas, belonged to the family of coarse, uninhalable burley tobaccos and were smoked in pipes and cigars. With Bright tobacco, it was now possible to make a smoking product which became known as cigarettes - literally, small cigars - that were inhalable, compact, exceptionally portable, and smokable all day long. Bright tobacco was also cheap to grow.

These first "inhaling cigars" were hand rolled by smokers, but from the first, the tobaccos assumed brand names.

Initially, people had a tendency to associate tobaccos with their place of purchase or, in some cases, the part of the country or even a special piece of land where they were grown. Branding happens to be a natural occurrence that consumers themselves seek out, first in differentiating the taste qualities of a product and then out of a spontaneous need to establish a personal and psychologically satisfying association with the product.

Wine is a good example of spontaneous branding. Even though it is an arcane business to the outsider, with few brands ever advertised, wines have always been branded with estate names and have become famous through word of mouth, articles, and published guides. Certain labels, such as Lafite and Margaux, have acquired a brand status by virtue of their stellar quality. Yet at every level consumers are making brand decisions of their own from the very coarse description, "French and about $10" to the predictable qualities of advertised brands like Corvo and Riunite. Even with drugs, which have no packaging or advertising at all, branding has always been part of it, from the psychedelic names given to acid like "Purple Haze" in the sixties to exotic names given to new strains of marijuana today, including Acapulco Gold, Superskunk, and White Whidow.

The difference is that once great marketing forces are thrown in behind brands their images themselves become an important property. The success of

Riunite and Bolla is closely tied to the images that these products have evolved with good advertising. It is not enough to put these marketing resources behind any brand; there has to be a certain level quality but, more than that, the key is finding the right image or perceptual value to which millions of otherwise uninterested people will respond. The lack of consistency of wine from a particular estate has always complicated the choice of wines. Oenophiles like to appear knowledgeable and adventurous. Yet broad information can be drawn from peoples' wine selections because there is usually a pattern. They could be Napa Valley lovers selecting Stag's Leap and Kendall-Jackson as their preferred brands, or they could go by Wine Spectator recommendations, or try their own discoveries, which will soon tag them to a particular price, locality, or name strategy. As always, their intention will be to find a good wine but within these selections, there will always be something that defines them that confirms or enhances their status as a selector of wines.

What makes cigarettes unique - and almost the polar opposite of wine selections - is that once people decide on a brand they stick with it. They rarely try showing off with other brands, like venturing out for Balkan Sobranies instead of their usual Marlboro. Unlike wine, the cigarette brand is too much a part of their personality to be dallied with. Once they have learnt to draw energy from the brand of the cowboy, they generally want no other.

The fact that the smoking public not only seeks out but clings to cigarette branding is the main reason why, once cigarettes have been established in the public mind, advertising is no longer as crucial to smokers as advertising might be to other products like soap or margarine. Aside from the fact that smokers are addicted - and advertising is not going to change that one way or the other - they are very loyal to their particular brands. Smokers rarely brand-hop unless they trading down to save money nor are they tempted the way laundry detergent or consumers of breakfast cereals are by an ad for another brand, a new type of packaging, or even a special deal. That is why, once the brand myth has been established, the major purpose of the advertising is to recruit new smokers while trying to keep smoking acceptable before the public. As Marshall Blonsky, the symbol professor at the New School in New York, once said: "The brand is like the Cheshire Cat's smile; once you have the smile you don't need the cat any more." Even **Winston** found they could spark interest just by showing the partial name on their packs.

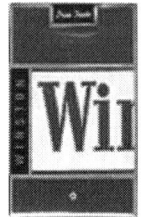

Certainly, tobacco companies are interested in getting smokers to switch, which is very hard to do, especially when, for the same effort they could go after initiating smokers - or starters, as they are known in the business - who have the potential to stick to a brand for many more years to come. But when tobacco companies do try getting people to switch, their only weapons other than price is their potential to exploit some psychological value as expressed in the mythic story of the brand. There are not that many really compelling archetypes which explains why smokers, other than the ones saving money with cut-price, generic brands which are usually sly knock-offs of major brands anyway, are rarely seen with new brands. Since the image is the most important element, it is quite likely that if tobacco companies had to choose between giving up advertising or giving up their individual brand identity and only use so-called gravestone advertising that has no image appeal, they would quickly forgo the advertising and hang on to the brand; that is, its name, its packaging, and the accumulated meaning of all its advertising and marketing to date.

It is an interesting phenomenon that prior to the massive $25 billion settlement which added up to $5 a pack in cigarette taxes, the profits of tobacco companies in recent years have soared in spite of the fact that the universe of U.S. smokers is shrinking. One reason is that without the TV medium tobacco companies can spend less on advertising and still reach their customers who, once persuaded, tend to stay with their brand. In general, tobacco companies would prefer to have the right to advertise. But they could also live without it because the biggest brands are so well established that they no longer have to evangelize vast numbers of the population - the thing advertising is best suited for. It is much more cost effective for them to market their product to a known segment of the marketplace that is smoker-friendly. Putting out brand messages in candy stores and gas stations and in other places where people do the ordinary business of their lives is by now the most efficient way to reach their target market.

In certain ways, established tobacco companies would gladly forgo advertising. The cost of national advertising in this adversarial climate may not even be worthwhile for the big **Players,** who they realize that using just the minimum advertising necessary to keep their name out there is enough to keep out newcomers while saving them a fortune in marketing costs. In many respects, the industry's fight for the right to advertise is as much about appearing a decent citizen as it is about maintaining a climate of acceptance for their products. They are well aware that drugs sell well without advertising and so could this product also.

Interestingly, the power of tobacco companies over the media and their ability to discourage them from running anti-smoking articles in the nineteen seventies and eighties and then their sudden loss of control in the nineties tells us a great deal about the relationship between who is buying the ads and the stories that media carry. There has always been a virtual blackout on cigarette stories in print publications, including newspapers, as long as cigarette companies advertised in them. But when the tobacco companies voluntarily ceased advertising on TV in 1970 there was still relatively little tobacco coverage on TV until the nineties because the tobacco companies had bought up breweries and food companies. If a TV network ran a negative story on Virginia Slims, or merely pointed out that more women were suffering from tobacco-related ailments because they were smoking in increasing numbers, the networks might face the ire of Kraft Foods or Miller Beer. Likewise, if Camel came under attack at one network then there was a distinct possibility of Nabisco ads moving to another network.

At one point, because tobacco companies like Reynolds, Philip Morris and Lorillard had become food and beer conglomerates that could express annoyance by withholding any number of ads from the media, anti-smoking groups became terrified at the prospect of free speech being stifled by commercial speech. Philip Morris' sponsorship of the tour of the Constitution in the early nineties was, to the health advocates, the ultimate insult, since it was supposed to show Philip Morris' support of the Bill of Rights even though the company had effectively stifled the First Amendment, thanks to their chilling effect on the media.

Two things worked to change that. One was the sheer health of network TV and its relative lack of advertising inventory. It became a seller's market and the big tobacco/food companies lost their leverage. Even if they threatened to pull their ads, there were other advertisers ready to take their space. A more subtly compelling explanation was that suddenly a product category emerged that competed directly with cigarettes: smoke cessation products like **Nicoderm** and **Nicotrol,** which the FDA had cleared for over-the-counter sale.

Suddenly, the power of tobacco companies to reward and punish networks was matched by the advertising power of drug giants like Smith Kline Beecham and McNeil Consumer Products. Almost overnight, network TV, which had long considered tobacco stories as ratings poison, was running special segments about the evils of second-hand smoke, the health effects of smoking, and the perfidy of the tobacco industry.

The power of companies who advertise is such that the future of cigarettes will likely become a battle between the "good" drug companies saving us from addiction and tobacco companies inventing less lethal ways to deliver nicotine. **Kraft Cheese** and **Nabisco** cookies have given way to **Claritin** and **Vioxx** ads and the balance of power has shifted. As we will see later, the paths will certainly cross and they may both end up competing to sell nicotine delivery products.

The net result for the first decade of the twenty first century is that the ability of the tobacco companies to influence society through advertising and its influence over commercial media has been substantially undermined. They continue to flourish anyway but they can no longer use the media against their critics. On the other hand, as far as the anti-smoking forces are concerned, the threat of banning advertising is no longer a choke point for the industry. Nowadays, the only real threat to tobacco sales - short of prohibition - would be the debranding of cigarettes. Commodity cigarettes would undermine the initiation value and would take the incentive away from mature companies like RJR and Philip Morris, that can be sued, to stay in the game. An industry would then be in the hands of small, fly-by-night companies who could not pay the legal damages and, in some cases, not even the taxes the big **Players** can pay.

Tobacco also has an uncanny ability to survive because it can take on many forms and different roles in society. When they first appeared as consumer items at the end of the nineteenth century, cigarettes were considered a godsend because, prior to World War I, most Americans chewed and then spat out their tobacco. Cigars were common, but women rarely smoked. Chewing tobacco and the brass spittoon, or in more dignified circles, the cuspidor, was a fixture on the floors of bars and restaurants for expectorating customers. At the same time, cigarettes were considered effeminate.

In the milestones of cigarette development it was the invention of the Bonsack cigarette-making machine in 1865 that introduced mass production and transformed a minor vice into a product of the industrial age. The giant industry we know today with all refinements of cigarette tobaccos, filters, mass marketing, psychological research and the major youth-oriented brand formulation of the nineteen fifties reflects the development of America's twentieth century industrial age.

The Bonsack machine made cigarettes economical to produce for the mass-market, but that market wasn't very interested for the first 50 years because cigars and chewing tobacco were the leading forms of consumption. Ironically, the biggest supporters of cigarettes were public health officials who saw them as salvation from the health hazards of widespread public spitting. In the early nineteen hundreds the New York City Health Department even issued a notice in support of cigarettes because a tuberculosis epidemic had caused the spitting of tobacco juice in to public cuspidors to be a disease carrier. As usual, however, the public wasn't much ready for what was "good" for them and they ignored cigarettes' health benefits at the time and continued to chew tobacco.

Even though there had been creeping acceptance of cigarettes in the early part of the twentieth century, the centralization of production had enabled a few companies to grow so big that eventually the tobacco trust was crushed under the wrath of Teddy Roosevelt. The end result, rather like the AT&T break-up in the nineteen eighties, produced a dominant player and many smaller competitors. In 1912 the break-up left American Tobacco, with its Lucky Strike brand, the major player, with several smaller companies, Lorillard, RJ Reynolds, Ligget & Myers created out of American Tobacco Trust's divested brands.

From a social and marketing perspective, it was World War I that put cigarettes on the map. Out in the trenches of Europe, the doughboys found their European counterparts happily smoking cigarettes without ever considering them a threat to their masculinity. The GIs soon borrowed this habit, which was fueled by the mostly free distribution of cigarettes with their food rations, so that when Johnny came marching home he was ready for cigarette smoking in a big way. In fact, he was gleefully hooked and he found his addiction widely encouraged by the then newly emerging phenomenon of the mechanized age - mass marketing.

While we do know that at first companies were satisfied with creating new brands on the basis of luck and intuition, it wasn't too long before the formal art of psychoanalysis was introduced into the game. That happened in 1922 when Edward L. Bernays, the man who many consider to be the father of public relations, was retained by American Tobacco's flamboyant president, George Washington Hill, to work on the Lucky Strike account.

G.W. Hill is usually considered to have been the model for the tyrant in Frederic Wakeman's "The Hucksters," a 1946 novel which became a movie with Clark Gable and Sidney Greenstreet. Hill wasn't totally sold on Bernays' ability when it came to marketing cigarettes; he only retained him as a way to keep him out of the hands of his competitors at RJ Reynolds. Bernays' reputation was such that Hill felt it would have been a blow against his company if anyone else had hired him. According to Bernays in "Biography of Idea," Hill had no real desire to use him and Bernays, who was related both to Sigmund Freud's wife, Anna Bernays, and more distantly to Freud himself, brought psychoanalysis into the tobacco industry as a result of his conscientiousness and this tobacco executive's paranoia.

In spite of what should have been a sinecure, Bernays was keen to give his client his money's worth and quickly set about earning his annual retainer of $25,000. His first accomplishment was persuading Hill to let him hire a psychoanalyst to put cigarettes on the couch, which he did once he had told Hill that it would cost nothing more than the price of an hour's consultation.

What Bernays recognized early in the game was that cigarettes, more than anything else, are a perceptual product because they have no physical benefits other than the creation of psychological and physical dependence. He also realized that cigarettes had a close relationship to the central fears or desires of people in a society. The result, as we will see, is that Bernays not only made his mark by introducing depth psychology to smoking but also helped accelerate its acceptance among women when his consultations with Brill identified the link between emancipation and smoking. As long as the relationship between cigarette image and psychology was established, it became possible for the astute marketer to tap the culture for successful brands.

To assess the importance of the image, it is worth considering that many blind taste tests have shown that smokers can't tell one brand from another. Once they are aware of the brand, however, their perception of the taste is modified instantly. The truth about these tests is that the people are usually asked to smoke just one cigarette of each brand. But if they could smoke several of each brand they would have a better chance of identifying them. Smokers do have powers of taste discrimination; it just takes a lot of puffing and it is limited to fairly simple factors such as whether the brand is "wet" or "dry." It is a rare smoker that can identify a brand the way a wine expert might detect an estate from a blind taste. Yet a smoker is a great deal less likely to deviate from his or her regular brand than an oenophile is. The reason is that smokers are not inhaling the flavor as much as they are absorbing the image.

When it comes to the image, it is worth taking into account what a tobacco executive once said about cigarette pack images. In Chris Mullen's **Cigarette Pack Art** (St. Martin's Press, 1979), a Philip Morris executive is quoted as saying, "20 times a day you take out your pack - it must mean something." Since the packages of successful cigarettes rarely change - only the advertising gets an overhaul every two or three years - it certainly does mean something. The question is what does it mean and how do we make sense of it?

In the following chapters we will explore the basic language of cigarette brands. Their core appeals are relatively simple and the vocabulary of benefits promised by the leading tobacco brands require only some fairly obvious product knowledge and a little interpretive creativity to make sense of them. By looking at the background of the brand and taking guidance from the advertising in the way, perhaps, that ancient travelers followed the stars, we discover the mythical lay of the land in the name, while the symbols and design of the pack trace a map of the smoker's unconscious mind.

From this unique vocabulary we learn what magic Madison Avenue offers teens at that critical moment of growing up. From this language of benefits a new generation will have the ability to understand their own vulnerabilities and perhaps craft a new language of response.

CHAPTER 5: DEATH AND SEX AND CIGARETTES

Understanding the man - or woman - by the brand they smoke has many limitations when compared to more traditional personality tests. But the upside is that smokers are available for examination whenever they light up and their brand choice touches upon the two issues that go to the core of our existence: sex and death.

The sexual meaning of cigarettes was first identified by Dr. Brill in the nineteen twenties when Edward Bernays hired him for his skeptical client, George Washington Hill of American Tobacco. Hill's major preoccupation at the time was how could American Tobacco sell Lucky Strikes to women?

Smoking had always been frowned upon by women in good society. But Hill wanted to expand the market for his already successful brand and had felt intuitively that there was a relationship to smoking and women's growing emancipation. He was groping about for a way of using this idea of freedom to sell them on Lucky Strikes.

Being a member, as it were, of the psychoanalytic movement, Bernays took great pleasure in hiring Dr. Brill, Freud's first American translator, to put smoking on the couch for his client. According to Bernays' Memoirs, "Biography of an Idea," Brill sallied forth identifying the unconscious significance of cigarettes as that of a phallic symbol, which was likely to be interpreted by women as a torch of freedom. His first report, which was textbook Freud and eerily ahead of its time, went as follows:

"Some women regard cigarettes as symbols of freedom. Smoking is a sublimation of oral eroticism; holding a cigarette in the mouth excites the oral zone. It is perfectly normal for women to want to smoke cigarettes. Further, the first woman who smoked probably had an excess of masculine components and adopted the habit as a masculine act. But today the emancipation of women has suppressed many of their feminine desires. More women now do the same work as men do. Many women bear no children; those who do have fewer children. Feminine traits are masked. Cigarettes, which are equated with men, become torches of freedom."

That a psychoanalyst would see a phallic reference in a cigarette is almost predictable. But that doesn't make it any less valid and the theme is an enduring one. It recurs in any number of ways in any number of campaigns. In general, it explains the element of power and compensation that people find in smoking. It even helps us understand why people often adopt smoking as a support device while they are engaged in the migration from a repressed to a liberated environment. It also explains the attraction that some people have for cigarettes even though they do not ultimately become smokers. As we will see, getting hooked is part of the allure, although few people expect to get hooked for life.

Brill was to elaborate on his analysis of smoking in a later report. Hill had hired him to analyze a new ad campaign for Lucky Strike about which he had nagging doubts. The campaign centered around a woman who was shown offering two men a cigarette. Brill advised strongly against it:

"Two people should appear, one man and one woman. That is life. Nor should a woman offer two men a package of cigarettes. The cigarette is a phallic symbol, to be offered by a man to a woman. Every normal man or woman can identify with such a message."

Like any symbol, there is a delicate balance between the inherent meaning of an object and what we want it to mean. A cigarette can stand for a number of meanings, ranging from the male principle, a sense of sexual allure, to a crucible of the tensions between the sexes. While it takes a certain amount of insight to trace the links between the smoker and his or her feelings, there are some very obvious clues in situations. When women smoke obviously male cigarettes like Marlboro or **Winston** or when men smoke women's brands like Virginia Slims and More, something important is being conveyed.

In essence, when you look at sex in cigarettes you are really looking at an emotional polarity: on the one hand a smoker is consuming what is essentially a pacifier for grown-ups and on the other hand he or she is displaying a symbol of power. How do you reconcile a product that is both a wishful penis and an adult pacifier?

It is acceptable for a father to smoke a cigar after the birth of a child because it is a symbolic demonstration of his virility. It is easy to tell the difference between someone following a ritual and a person who needs that emotional support. But how can we tell whether that person is trying to recapture childhood or add imaginary testosterone to his character? We can only look at the smoker and ask where he or she stands on that scale and determine whether they are using it predominantly for one purpose or the other. Are they seeking the "paradise lost" of their early years or are they posing with aggression? And since most people employ a combination of both at the same time, what really are its dynamics - do they recede when they puff on the cigarette and then surge when they exhale? Do they handle it for comfort or as a power accessory?

The dark side of smoking is the willing assumption of ill-health and eventually death in pursuit of pleasure. While it may seem like the ultimate form of self-punishment, in reality, it works as the ultimate form of self-control so smokers can also be graded on this basis: are they smoking to control themselves, which is an arguably constructive purpose, or is it to punish themselves? Again, it is more often than not a combination of the two and you would want to look at its dynamics. People who smoke are aware of the self-destructive side of smoking and that they are forming a relationship with it. Although they may deny ever thinking about it, they have obviously given some thought to its role and its consequence in their lives.

In fact, Ernest Dichter, in another moment of public openness not often seen in this business, once stated in a Forbes Magazine article in 1966 that he began his research with the assumption that "smokers really want to kill themselves." Health officials are prone to describe smoking as former Surgeon General Koop once did: "a form of slow-motion suicide." But smokers are more likely to feel fatalistic about it, saying that it is just a kind of lottery or even a less drastic form of Russian roulette. If they take a more positive view, they might just be saying, "Smoking may be killing me but since I am going to die anyway, at least now I control my ability to live or die."

It would take some digging or at least a very subtle eye to determine the attitude a smoker has about his or her habit. But if you could determine that, you would find out a lot about smokers inner drives. For example, the more fatalistic the smoker feels about his habit the more likely he is to be a follower, while the more he feels he "controls" his ability to live or die, the more he is likely to be a leader. In any case, no one who smokes is unaware of the risks they are taking and they will all have evolved some form of internal justification. Because they are indulging in this habit for very high stakes with a high degree of awareness, their brand selections are very meaningful.

Does that suggest there is a sex and death index? And if one existed, could we measure this in smokers? The answer is that to some extent we can tell from the intensity with which someone smokes just how much they are willing to put themselves at risk. If they savor the cigarette or treat at it with a sense of disdain, then we can make a rough judgment as to how reckless they will be or how far they are willing to go in pursuit of pleasure. There may be other cues, such as an excess of hand motions during smoking, which can suggest compensation or masking of the smoker's real emotions. If you can determine what smokers are most willing to put themselves at risk for, you will be able to uncover the key issues of their lives: their inner emotional problems, the crosses they bear, or just what bothers them most.

Having power over life is what gives cigarettes their "spirit power." People smoke in full knowledge of cigarettes' deadliness but they do it because they think smoking is taking care of something worse than the obvious prospect of death. For example, smoking might give a very lonely smoker a sense of companionship or a means of quashing her rage. Or it could be a source of strength or a consolation for lacking strength. Often you can tell that from the way smokers show possession of their packs - do they always keep them on their persons or do they leave them lying about? The point is to determine the relationship the smokers develop with their brand. First, however, you need to know a little about the brands, starting with the most important brand of the post-World War II era, the brand that has defined success in a cigarette brand: Marlboro.

CHAPTER 6: HOW MARLBORO BECAME A MAN....

The meaning of the brand wasn't really understood until the nineteen fifties, when the new Marlboro burst in on the scene. This was the first time a brand was created out of extensive psychological research and not just happenstance. There was a clear intent by the creators to reach out to a mythic dimension and in doing so, Philip Morris, the manufacturer, produced one of advertising's most enduring icons.

Back in the 'thirties, when Philip Morris had first used a central character in its advertising it had been something clever like the bell hop, Johnny Roventini, who did the "Call for Philip Morris!" campaign. Back then, his rationale was to associate the brand with fine hotels and the idea that the bellhop made you, the smoker seem important (a call for you!). Of course, his clear, calling voice implied that cigarettes improved his vocal chords.

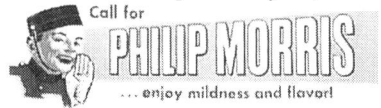

When Johnny the bellhop went on to become famous in his own right, it was a pleasant surprise for the company. People weren't actually supposed to identify with him - just the hotel society he served so he was hardly the hero in the true sense of the word. There may well be an argument that he represented the joker or wizard, the likable character in Jungian psychology. The joker, who may also create trouble, is often considered able to lead people to higher knowledge. This is not a mere abstraction -- there is rarely a Disney film made without a likable, slightly zany character who helps save the day. He could be R2D2 in **Star Wars**, the mongoose in **The Jungle Book** or Wilson in **Home Improvement**. Whatever the deeper reason though, he was popular.

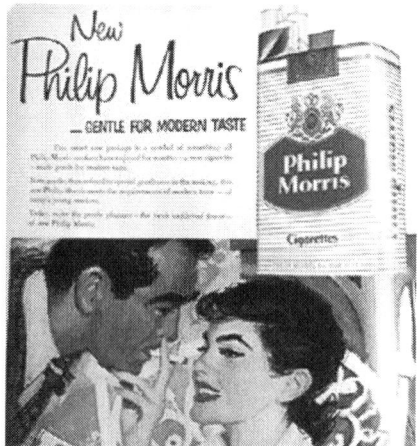

Even though Roventini was a hero of sorts and Philip Morris must have been impressed with the power of a compelling character, his days were numbered once the cancer scare first hit in the late 'forties. That was when cancer researcher Alton Ochsner noted the correlation between smoking and lung cancer in a 1939 paper published in Surgery, Gynecology and Obstetrics. He and Dr. Michael DeBakey reported that, "In our opinion the increase in smoking with the universal custom of inhaling is probably a responsible factor, as the inhaled smoke, constantly repeated over a long period of time, undoubtedly is a source of chronic irritation to the bronchial mucosa." The only response the company and their ad agency, the now defunct Milton

Biow organization, could come up with was the campaign: "New Philip Morris: Made Gentle for You" and "Gentle for Modern Tastes." That proved hard to reconcile with this cocky little fellow with a big voice and so the brand faded.

It was after the failure of this campaign that Philip Morris decided to take an entirely different approach with a new filter cigarette they, like others in the industry were planning. Viceroy had introduced the first filter cigarette in 1951 but it had been a tepid seller with a lackluster campaign by Rosser Reeves, who later became a legend in advertising by introducing the idea of the Unique Selling Proposition, the USP. The USP here was the filter but the campaign psychology was all wrong: "When You think About It You Smoke Viceroy." In his 1961 biography, **Reality in Advertising**, Reeves said he never asked the customer to think about anything again after that. Smoking is not an intellectual experience and if you were to really think about it, you would not want to smoke.

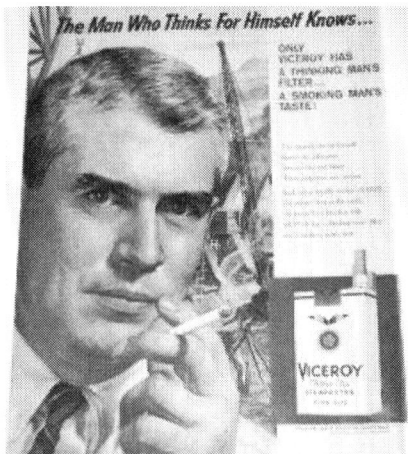

Nevertheless, Philip Morris executives realized that filters were the future and in order to make them acceptable and overcome their "wimp" image they would have to come up with a heroic, masculine figure. Initially, they were just after a stereotype of a certain kind of working class male - easy-going and macho. But later, as we will see, it all came together in the Western archetype we are still enamored with today.

We do know that although $200,000 was spent on research, and the company appeared to know exactly what **it** were looking for, Marlboro's success did involve a degree of serendipity. The cowboy was not originally intended to be the leading man but just one of many macho "spokestypes." Initially, the imagery produced by the newly hired Leo Burnett ad agency in Chicago was only macho in a general sense. According to reports in Fortune magazine, the type they were after was compiled from profiles psychologists had made at of an ideal male at the time. The typical model, who might be described as appearing relaxed and macho, was beefy in a laid-back way, and was shown in the profile with pictures of him fishing from a boat, wearing a relaxed smile and sporting a tattoo.

to Chicago on the Twentieth Century Limited and had a meeting with Leo Burnett, the founder of the advertising agency that bears his name. 'Here's your ad,' he said and he threw it on the table. 'Says it right there. New from Philip

Morris. The cowboy, a symbol of masculine virility. Filter, flavor, flip-top box.'"

That is of course a romanticized version because we know that the first ad was not a cowboy but someone looking more like a lifeguard. We also have early ads showing mechanics, detectives, and young, likable punk types. While the cowboy was used in the ads, it took a few years before he was isolated as the single Marlboro Man symbol. But it does seem clear that from the very first they knew what they were looking for. It just took a while before they realized the cowboy was it.

To begin with, Marlboro wasn't a new brand. In fact it was one of those very rare things in marketing - a drastic repackaging of a pre-existing brand. The original Marlboro, which first appeared in the nineteen twenties, had been a woman's cigarette that was not sold in regular outlets but only in restaurants and beauty parlors at a premium. Some of the slogans used to advertise it were "Mild as May" and "Ivory Tips Protect Your Lips."

The old Marlboro was never very suc-
cessful and at various times Philip Morris tried marketing techniques that would seem mildly bizarre today. For example, to emphasize its mildness, they ran ads with pictures of a mother and her baby declaring the brand, "Mild as May." In the early nineteen forties they tried bringing out a version with lipstick-painted tips. This was supposed to solve a problem women had with their lipstick rubbing off on their cigarettes. Back then, lipstick did not stay on as well as it does today, so it had to be reapplied throughout the day, especially if the wearer smoked. It even became a Hollywood cliché, with vampy actresses teasing sex appeal from putting on lipstick after a smoke. The Marlboro tips were an innovative attempt to solve this problem. Unfortunately, it was discovered that while most lipstick is red, there are many subtle shades of red and the Marlboro red tips tended to clash with their regular colors.

While Marlboro's sales were languishing, a series of events taking place in the 'forties and 'fifties had executives at Philip Morris deeply concerned. It began officially in 1945 when Dr. Alton Ochsner of the American Cancer Society announced that there was a link between smoking and cancer. A number of studies later appeared, giving credence to his observation, and by the early nineteen fifties, enough of this had been picked up by the press to give it the name "cancer scare."

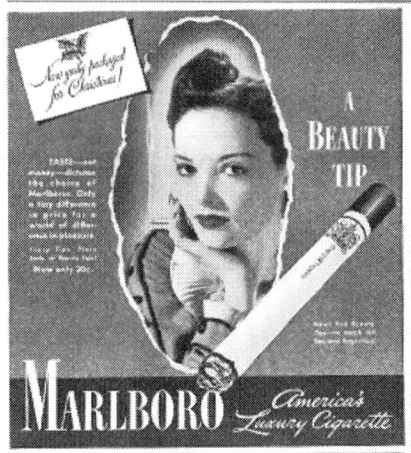

In public, the industry's response was to roll out the kinds of campaigns that almost earned the Cipollone estate its $400,000: "More Doctors Smoke Camel Than Any Other Cigarette," "Not a Cough In A Carload" (Old Gold), and "The Throat-Tested Cigarette" (Philip Morris). In private, though, they began to think of more effective long-term strategies. There were rumors going round that the R.J Reynolds tobacco company of **Winston-Salem**, North Carolina, had begun working on a new brand of cigarettes that would address this health problem. At the same time there was a general realization in the industry that they were marketing to a nation that had fought two significant foreign wars within the same generation - World War II and Korea. Cigarettes had not only sold exceptionally well during those periods but the country had welcomed the kinds of patriotic ads that accompanied them, such as "Lucky Strike Green Goes To War" and the Camel series about bomber pilots who calmed their nerves with cigarettes. Cigarettes were so popular that they had been rationed in wartime England while in the U.S. they were declared a strategic crop by President Roosevelt. Marketers in the nineteen fifties remembered well those profitable years and the inherent magic of the nation's war memories.

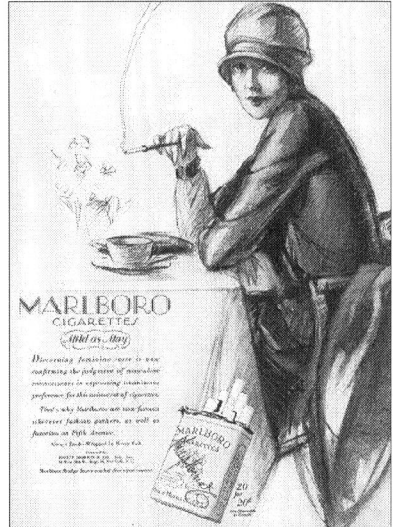

At the same time, it was obvious to the best minds in the industry that they had to respond directly to the health scare. At Philip Morris, before the cancer scare had erupted in the media, Joseph Cullman III noticed a sales increase in Parliament, an unadvertised brand sold only in exclusive tobacco stores. When he asked around, he was told that doctors had been alerted by privately published studies to the possible ill effects of smoking. As a result, they were recommending Parliaments to their patients on the theory that their cardboard mouthpieces with filters made them safer. Introduced in the late thirties, Parliament's filters were made from wads of cotton but they were not very efficient, clogging easily and making the cigarettes difficult to smoke.

The breakthrough in the industry was the development of cellulose filters which were capable of reducing the apparent tar content while allowing the smoke to pass through freely. But when these filters appeared in the brand Viceroy, the public seemed to view them as effeminate, so shrewd executives realized the need for imagery that would make filters acceptable. They also understood, thanks to researchers like Dichter, that health claims in cigarettes were a bad way to sell cigarettes. Dichter called these health claims "a form of industry suicide" because they only exacerbated fears and created the impression that the industry was caving in to the health critics. What they really needed a new image: Arabia was out and simple American folk art like Lucky Strike, with its roots in the gold rush days, was passé: They needed to find a new frontier.

"You're like part of the family, Doctor!"

MORE DOCTORS SMOKE CAMELS THAN ANY OTHER CIGARETTE

CAMELS Costlier Tobaccos

The process behind finding the names of the two new filter cigarettes that were about to appear on the market is mired in secrecy and glossed over in published reports about the creation of these brands. It is clear, however, that these names were a product of their times. In an era still intoxicated with the glory of World War II, it should come as no surprise that brands which resonated with the names and characters of the war years would have a special appeal.

As the story goes, by 1954 it was the R,J. Reynolds company that was expected to come out with the first filtered, male-oriented cigarette. They had made early announcements and the industry was anxiously anticipating their move. Unexpectedly, the much smaller Philip Morris Company pre-empted Reynolds by coming out first with their macho, filtered brand called Marlboro. Reynolds, on the other hand, was taking its time with a new product called **Winston**. But other than Philip Morris pulling an end run on Reynolds, was there a relationship between the two brands?

Superficially, Reynolds had named **Winston** for the first half of its hometown, **Winston-Salem**. That is the official story, but the reason the name *sounded* so good is because it rode on the coattails of one of World War II's grand heroes, **Winston** Churchill. The fact that Churchill wasn't just a hero but a *foreign* one didn't hurt in this case either. He was an ally, spoke English, and was both old and foreign enough that he could not cloud his reputation the way, for example, General Douglas MacArthur did in Korea. Unlike MacArthur, Churchill was a great cigar smoker - a very masculine image – rather than a pipe smoker, which is usually considered ruminative. To make matters worse, MacArthur smoked a corn-cob pipe, which may be folksy but also says country bumpkin. Churchill even came out looking better than FDR, who used cigarette holders, which were considered effeminate.

The other link between **Winston**'s pack and the benighted Sir **Winston** Churchill was the symbol of a crown over the description line, "King Size." Eventually, after 25 years on the market, Reynolds dropped that crown and replaced it with an American eagle, which, interestingly enough, became an element of growing importance in their ads. It is worth noting that **Winston**, which has this association with a great orator, tends to attract a garrulous person as opposed to Marlboro, which is part of a more laconic, John Wayne tradition.

According to RJ Reynolds' 1984 secret strategic market research documents released in the Minnesota lawsuit, **Winston** became identified with the kind of masculinity that people associated with the unpopular Vietnam war, and the brand suffered accordingly, losing sales to young people,

The report stated: "**Winston** may have lost popularity among younger adult smokers because changes in the external environment made **Winston** less in tune with both the demographics and the mindset of the nineteen sixties than it had been in the 1950s. Its large number of older smokers may have contributed by linking the brand to the 'establishment'.....**Winston**'s light-hearted...campaign fit well with the mindset of the 50s *(i.e., Winston Tastes Good Like a Cigarette Should)*, but did not fit as well with the rising tide of intense younger adult rebels as Marlboro did in the 1960s.....[and] may have become less attuned to the changing younger adult mindset of the 1960s. In the era of Vietnam, campus riots, and the Chicago Seven, it seems likely that Marlboro's intense, unsmiling cowboy was a better fit."

Back in the fifties, Philip Morris realized it had a kind of titled asset of its own, one which went on to represent the fighting knight and modern keeper of the chivalric code, the cowboy. In their case it was a languishing woman's brand called Marlboro, which is really an Americanized version of Marlborough. As it happens, this brand had a close titular relationship to **Winston** Churchill who had become known for a revival of his own: the family name of his ancestor, the First Duke of Marlborough, who had beaten the French under Louis XIV at the Battle of Blenheim but later fell out of political favor and was discredited by the crown. Churchill had written a passionate and highly publicized biography defending the Duke and attempted to regain the Marlborough title, which had been taken away from his family. With the knowledge that a brand with a militaristic tradition like **Winston** was on its way, how could Philip Morris resist a name like Marlboro?

Curiously, at around the same time the Japanese were getting ready to bring out a filtered cigarette of their own. The pack was designed by the famous Raymond Loewy, who was responsible for the U.S. Post Office's flying eagle, the Exxon logo, and the redesign of the Lucky Strike package during World War II. This time Loewy was not hired to do a package design with a war connection. Indeed, he seemed like a strange choice altogether. Perhaps it was a gesture of conciliation then that the Japanese, still recovering from a war they lost, hired the man who did so much to change the look of America to design the packaging for a new brand called Peace.

One thing we are sure of is that Philip Morris was well aware of the importance of the military iconography, because we have a record of the research process. The guiding light behind Marlboro was a wartime naval officer and future chairman of Philip Morris, George Weissman, whose fascination with the military was summarized by the message on the cigarette box: "Veni. Vidi. Vici."

It has been reported that the Marlboro design was one of the most researched in history. The $200,000 Philip Morris spent on research was such a huge sum at the time that they publicized it the way Hollywood studios do with movie star's salaries. The design was handled by a leading graphics artist of the time, Frank Gianinoto, and it was heavily researched by Louis Cheskin, who was later to become quite famous because of his appearance in Vance Packard's advertising exposé, **The Hidden Persuaders**.

HOW TO PREDICT WHAT PEOPLE WILL BUY
by LOUIS CHESKIN

Louis Cheskin, Director of Color Research Institute, and George Weissman, Vice President of Philip Morris, reviewing ocular measurements and field tests of Philip Morris and Marlboro packages.

The Marlboro Man

Cheskin was a color and symbol researcher who had started out working in the Chicago school system. After several frustrating years of trying to persuade the system of the educational value of color psychology and art, he went into business for himself. He had already published little-known books in the nineteen forties, including **Living with Art** and **Colors -- What They Can Do For You**, and that lent him credibility as a new kind of perceptual researcher.

Cheskin's basic tools were a high speed projector called a tachistoscope that flashed an image on the screen for a split second, an eye-tracking machine that followed the subject's eyeballs as they read, and a

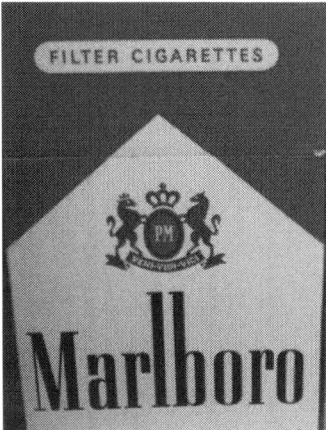

pupillometer that measured their emotional response according to the dilation of their pupils. After the tachistoscope flashed an image on a screen for a split second, Cheskin would then ask his subjects which elements they could remember so as to get a sense of the strongest element in an ad or design. He would use the eye-tracking machine to see how their eyes saccaded, or followed the ad. The pupillometer, which was often used in conjunction with the eye-tracking machine, could indicate the extent of the viewer's emotional response by measuring the dilation of the pupils. With this bag of tricks he could measure the feelings of smokers exposed to the various design elements involved in the new Marlboro package.

In describing the research in his book, **How to Predict What People Will Buy**, Cheskin said he found the response to the red and white colors predictably strong. But it was the crest he found most important because once it was removed, approval of the design dropped significantly. What was in that crest? Besides the "Veni.Vidi.Vici." inscription, the red banner at the top of the box gave it the appearance of an inverted ribbon. Then there was the pack itself -- a flip-top box that gave it a smart, ironed look. In other words, there was a combination of elements designed to resemble a medal.

The pack itself was an anomaly. Even going back as far as the original **Lucky Strike** and **Camel**, the typical American cigarette came in a soft pack. European brands are usually sold in a box, or among the rich, in small, ornate tins. The original woman's **Marlboro** came in a soft pack. But the new **Marlboro** appeared in something called the "crush proof" box which was supposed to protect the cigarettes. Even though brands like **Kent** and **Luckies** have used this package too, none has succeeded with it the way **Marlboro** has. Today, **Marlboro** is the only top-selling male brand where the hard packs outsell the soft.

So what's in a pack? Americans love a soft-pack for the same reason they enjoy a casual lifestyle. In Europe, where tradition

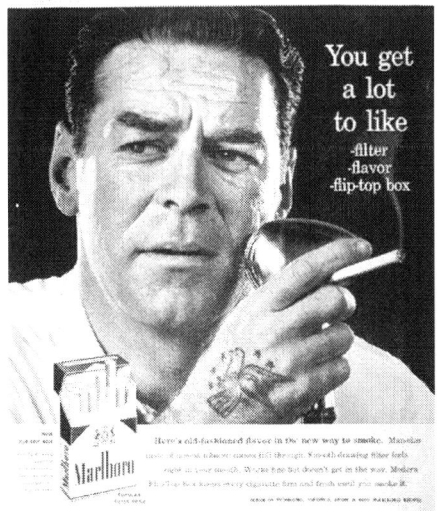

is a significant part of people's lifestyles, the hard pack reflects the needs of a more formal, stylized culture. It is the pack that holds and protects their stash – their daily spirit food. On an individual level, we can even make a judgment on pack choice: a more brittle or protective personality might go for the hard pack and a more flexible or easy-going personality for the soft pack. But if hard packs don't normally belong here, how did the hard pack become the container of choice among smokers identifying with **Marlboro's** easy-going macho stereotype?

As it happens, the hard pack is just one more element of **Marlboro's** militaristic tradition. It became the norm for **Marlboro** because men keep their cigarettes in their pockets – if they can, in their shirt pockets. That means every time they take out a cigarette and snap their pack shut they would be returning them to their shirt pockets if they could, just as if they were snapping a medal to their chest.

But another part of **Marlboro's** success depended on a certain bond it was able to make with its smokers at a very intimate level. In its world, it is a perfect example of a Madison Avenue-created totem that taps into tribal culture as effectively as Walt Disney has done with European folk culture.

When Philip Morris rolled out their introductory campaign for this new brand, it featured men with tattooed hands. This was a long, long time before tattoos became as prevalent as they are today. While mildly shocking at the time, the tattoos were significant for doing more than emphasizing the hands and beefy arms of the models; they were telling a multi-leveled story. At one level, the calculation behind the tattoos was obvious: they were temporary tattoos so the middle classes, in the days when tattoos were *not* in fashion, were reassured that something truly vile had not just occurred in their favorite magazines. Since the tattoos could be removed at any time, it also suggested that smoking was not an addiction but could as easily be stopped at any time and acted against any suggestion of bodily disfigurement and the permanent dangers of smoking.

The typical advertising textbooks say that in 1954, the idea of a tattoo just matched the times. Johnny was coming home from Korea just as he had done nine years before from Japan and Europe. He would have come into contact with foreign, often primitive cultures. Having a tattoo in the service was considered a legitimate ritual mark of acceptance within a warrior group. But the advertising still created a genuine sense of shock at the time. To deflect it, they made the models look as friendly as possible; after all, juvenile delinquents and youth gangs were just then being recognized as a social problem and tattoos proved to be very attractive to these subcultures.

Marlboro's enduring success was more than just the sum of its parts. It grew successful because it had struck a chord at a much deeper, unconscious level where it tapped memories that bind us to our tribal past. In the context of its times, the **Marlboro Man** entered the market by replaying a primitive initiation ceremony of danger and acceptance that remains the secret ingredient of its success to this day.

Primitive cultures generally rely on initiation and war to separate their boys from the girls. Prior to their coming-of-age, in most tribes, there is relatively little formal separation between the sexes. At the beginning of puberty or adolescence, the boys are usually required to undergo some form of an initiation that generally involves an act of bravery - sometimes the killing of a beast or even a man. When that has been accomplished, the young male is given an initiation mark usually involving some form of scarification or disfigurement. Among the darker-skinned peoples, like the Melanesians in Papua New Guinea and the aborigines in Australia, it is body paint; in Africa, it is a ritual face or body scarring called a cicatrix. In lighter-skinned societies like Polynesia, Greenland, Siberia, and even Japan, it is tattoos.

Philip Morris had created the tribal initiation equivalent with their package. In effect, the subliminal medal of the **Marlboro** pack and its tattoo advertising created the message that Philip Morris was offering an initiation device. It also told people a symbolic story, part of which was that the brand had undergone a gender change. By replacing the feminine white tips with cork-colored ones they were, in effect, saying they could make a man out of them while offering the reward of a ritual mark of acceptance. There is, after all, a reason why Marlboro remains the one "macho" brand women will smoke, while **Winston** is almost never smoked by women.

We know it took several years before Philip Morris recognized the cowboy as their prototypical American fighting man. Then, years later, they found that the **Marlboro Man's** mystique was so powerful that he could even survive his own disappearance. That was in the wake of the Surgeon-General's second report in 1974, which definitively linked smoking to cancer. It was considered dangerous on Madison Avenue to show people in cigarette ads since that risked heightening the smokers' awareness of

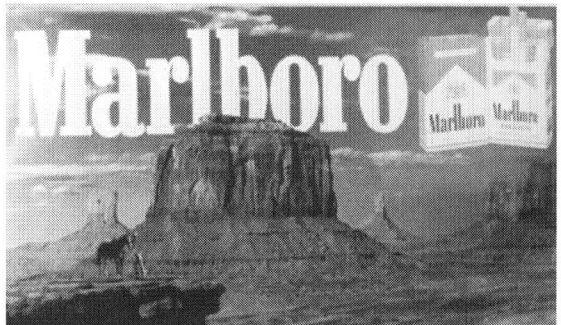

the dangers of tobacco. For this dark period, the **Marlboro Man** actually ceased to appear in his own ads.

The "me decade" of the seventies had made ads so personal there was the reasonable likelihood of smokers being turned off by humans in cigarette ads. What if people began to think about the health of the models? The prevailing wisdom was that having the old cowboy in the ad would seem to emphasize the personal message of cancer. Fortunately, he existed in a mythic landscape and they tried using the cowboy's lair instead of the cowboy with ads that spoke to smokers, along with: "Welcome to **Marlboro** Country." Curiously, this campaign succeeded not only because his arid stomping grounds were cancer-free but because the public also had a tendency to interpret the open, non-polluted country imagery as a health message. Nowadays, **Marlboro** often alternates between these two approaches of solitary man or pristine cowboy.

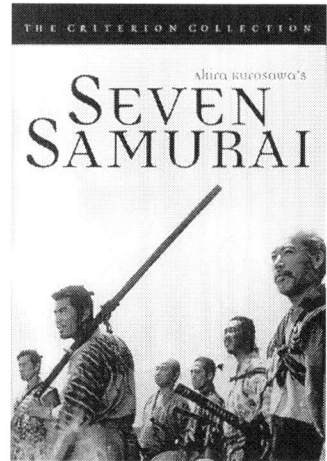

In retrospect, the use of the cowboy as a fighter archetype seems obvious and the initial groping that Philip Morris underwent before finding him seems hard to understand now. As we recognize today, the cowboy is the man who settled the West and then brought a rough law and order to it. Westerns had their own style of chivalry that was as well understood by its audience as the code of Medieval Knights or for that matter, the Samurai of Japan. Mythic fighting orders have a universal quality with the result that a 'fifties Japanese classic like Kurosawa's **The 7 Samurai**, could be transformed with relative ease by Hollywood into the classic western, **The Magnificent 7**. Except for the

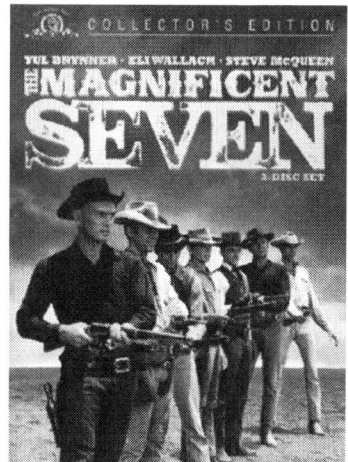

movie buffs, very few moviegoers knew they were really watching a Samurai story when Yul Brunner and crew rode into town with their guns a-blazing. Warrior myths exist in most cultures but Philip Morris was the first American company to identify the U.S. version in its purest form and put it in a box and let the public consume it.

To a generation returning from an unsatisfactory war, a 25¢ medal was a classic 'fifties example of taking an age-old concept, seemingly detached from its origins, and repackaging it for an industrial age. Instead of having to hunt or fight for the reward, one only had to work long enough to purchase it. If initiation is still an enduring fact of life among teens in primitive societies, what could be wrong with borrowing from that to appeal to teens in an *industrial* society?

A classic study in the nineteen seventies showed that 70% of a sample group of 100 white teenagers began their smoking with Marlboro. According to RJ Reynolds secret research documents, which were revealed in the breakthrough Minnesota lawsuit, "As a company Philip Morris held more than 60 percent of these 18 year old smokers in 1983 versus RJR's 15-20%." Since then, regardless of whose figures you work from, the percentage has remained steady - sometimes increasing. Among a similar study of a group of East Coast Hispanics the initiation brand of choice was **Newport**. Despite protestations to the contrary, cigarette companies need teenagers, or starters, very badly. The peak starting years for smokers is between the ages of 14 and 18. If the smokers haven't been initiated by the age of 21 they are not very likely to smoke. And if they haven't been initiated by the age of 25 they probably never will. Other studies have shown that the earlier one starts, the harder it is to quit. So as far as the tobacco industry is concerned, a teenage smoker represents the equivalent of a lifelong annuity while the older starter is much more likely to use their freedom of choice at some choice at some point and quit.

The continuing recognition of **Marlboro** as **the** American initiation brand can be attributed to a number of circumstances. True, the tattoo has long since disappeared but inasmuch as it has made an impression on the populace, the message has been passed down from parent to child and is part of the product's DNA. That is another thing studies have shown - that teens don't start because of advertising as much as they do from parental example and peer pressure. So, like any key message in culture, it has been passed down from generation to generation to the point where the meaning and consequences of **Marlboro** is understood by people without their necessarily knowing its origins.

The desire for a coming-of-age ritual that involves power, danger, and adequate symbols of acceptance is, in any case, strong enough that it is recognized by each coming generation. In the years before tobacco was widely believed to be a public health hazard, cigarettes were considered a natural accompaniment of young adulthood and they truly become a standard coming of age ritual. After the cancer scare, a brand had to address its dangers by playing up its allure. At first, **Marlboro** used tattoos on genial young men and then onto increasingly tougher men, ending up with today's grizzled cowboy. It is both ironic and only natural that 40 years later, as people grew to know more about cigarettes, a general interest in spirit power has led to a widespread interest in tattoos and other forms of visible body scarification. We have, in effect, moved from an era where our parents and grandparents once welcomed the cigarette as a worthy replacement to primitive ceremonies of adulthood that included body markings and scarification, to an era where they may replace or at least enhance smoking.

The phenomenon of teen culture that the cigarette companies have caught on to is this simple: physically, teenagers mature younger but they are forced to wait longer until they reach adulthood. Those are fertile years for experimentation and rebellion. At the same time, we have devised very few social channels that address that time of their lives in a positive way. Society offers no form of initiation. Nor do they provide the sense of induction into the secret body of knowledge of the "tribes" that is a key part of initiation ceremonies. In this cultural wasteland, cigarette brands have a siren appeal, and their allure to teens is a compelling mixture of danger, legality, independence, rebellion, and an opportunity to join a group as a brand member.

Smoking has assumed the role of a symbolic trial that starts out by being unpleasant. After coughing their way through the three weeks it takes to assume the habit, the teenagers also absorb the knowledge of its potential dangers. Under these circumstances, the health hazard is actually welcome because it tells them they have temporarily overcome it. Once the initiates are able to turn the discomfort of smoking into a form of pleasure, they are able to consider themselves having passed a test of adulthood. The idea is Nietschean: whatever doesn't kill me makes me stronger. The symbols on the pack and the blackening of one's lungs serve as the initiation mark.

Marlboro is still the leading choice because of its traditional references. It even contains the opening syllable "marl," suggesting a war wound, a kind of scar or symbol of toughness. Instead of killing a lion and then getting evidence of your prowess tattooed on your arms or carved into your chest, you only have to inhale **Marlboros**. The box even tells you can place it in your shirt pocket. Is it really a coincidence that the unofficial initiation ceremony of the Marines is the notorious "pinning" of newly graduated marines by tattooing a medallion on their chests.

When Ernest Dichter told Forbes Magazine that he began his research on the assumption that smokers were really trying to kill themselves, he went on to say that people chose 100 mm. cigarettes instead of the smaller king size because, "it is just like playing Russian Roulette with six barrels instead of five." (Actually, Dichter's math was wrong since the extra barrel would reduce the odds of dying. However, as Rosser Reeves pointed out in his biography of Dichter, people actually thought longer cigarettes like Pall Mall were safer because they provide more tobacco to "filter" the cigarette the smoke as it is being drawn in by the smoker.)

Is this slow motion suicide? Smokers may rationalize their habit as a form of self-control but at certain stages, particularly in their teen years, they definitely seek out danger for its own sake - and they want it quickly. The "Hidden Persuader" ad researcher, Pierre Martineau, first pointed this out as a general feature of smokers in his 1957 book, **Motivation In Advertising** (McGraw-Hill p. 33):

"Cigarette research reveals that masochistic tendencies (deliberately hurting oneself) are important features in smoking, but for the advertising man this leads nowhere."

That may arguably have been true in 1957. But in 1998, when tobacco executives themselves, as they did before Congress on January 29, 1998 referred to smoking as "risky" behavior that may indeed have a link to various kinds of heart and lung diseases, this information leads everywhere.

For teenagers, in particular, it means tapping into the awkward reality of reaching adulthood; it often means trying to discover a sense of their own mortality by flirting with the idea of death. To many teenagers, cigarettes are the first tangible evidence of having grown up, and cigarette advertising usually goes a long way to remind them of that.

The attitude of the tobacco companies to the mandatory health warnings on the packs also shows how ambiguous the issue of personal danger is when it comes to smoking. On the one hand, the warning indemnifies the companies from legal responsibility for health damage, so they could never again face a Cipollone-like judgment from post-1966 smokers. Then again, since smokers continue in full knowledge and in open complicity with the health hazard, cigarette executives can rationalize the ethics of the industry to their many workers. Profiting from an extremely lucrative industry is one thing, but with hundreds of thousands of people involved in the tobacco industry there is always the chance that *someone* would have a conscience. So industry workers have adopted a profound sense of helping people – that **by** providing their addicted customers what they so deeply want renders the din of controversy and the cries of moral outrage irrelevant.

If tobacco people are obliged to state in public that cigarettes are not harmful, it is strictly for PR purposes. They understand the value of having danger openly associated with their brands because it adds to its allure. More danger means a greater sense of control for the smoker and, for those who seek it, greater likelihood of death. Disclosing on the pack the possibility of death enhances the "spirit power" that is associated with the brand. Astute companies like Philip Morris understand, after having been involved in the sponsorship of religious art like "The Art of Vatican" and collections representing the Protestant denomination and the Jewish religion, that initiation rituals, like religious ceremonies, gain power from their association with and defiance of death. It is that seeming power over death, however temporary, however illusory, that is a major asset when it comes to a cigarette brand.

CHAPTER 7: ....AND WHAT KIND OF MAN?

When it comes to interpreting **Marlboro** smokers, you have to take into account some interesting anomalies. For all the apparent machismo of the brand, it is still by far the most popular man's brand to be smoked by women. Even the RJ Reynolds researcher Diane Burrows, whose papers appeared in the Minnesota court **proceedings**, agrees in a way that can only be described as politically correct for a corporate employee in the 'eighties: "As **Winston** lost its hold on the 18 year-old smoker market of the mid-1960s, its younger adult smokers dispersed to Saelm (sic) and Kool as well as to **Marlboro**. As with Pall Mall, **Winston**'s younger adult female smokers moved more quickly, leaving **Winston** overdeveloped among younger adult males for the first time." Translation: young women stopped smoking **Winston** - if they ever smoked them at all - just before Woodstock.

Nowadays, it is rare to find women smoking **Winston** or Lucky Strike. Camels have acquired a female clientele but that is a relatively new phenomenon related to the disarming quality of the cartoon Camel. The question is whether **Marlboro** became a unisex brand because of its transsexual history or because the cowboy myth is truly universal among genders as well as cultures.

A closer look at the package reveals that **Marlboro** has features that offer something for everyone. The world of cigarettes has its own vocabulary of graphic symbols that are modified in a kind of symbolic grammar. By understanding the basic message of each brand, it is possible to refine our knowledge of the user through an understanding of the "linguistic" rules of smoking. By taking into account the pack type, the cigarette length, the kind of filter as well as the smoker's style – that is, the way the cigarette is lit or put out, where the pack is kept and how it is discarded - we can often pinpoint the brand's meaning in a smoker's life.

The key elements of the **Marlboro** pack to take into account are the crest, its "roof" - the inverted v-shaped ribbon - the **Marlboro** logo with the narrow typeface, with the skinny "lb" in the name, and the hard pack itself.

If we were to create a profile of the **Marlboro** smoker as defined by the advertising message, it would go something like this: this is a person who responds to the martial aspect of the crest, and identifies with the lone cowboy image. Since these smokers are responding to a certain stereotype of a soldier, it is reasonable to expect that in general, they are instinctively responsive to orders but will also feel a need to temper that with some expression of irreverence. You would expect them to cherish signs of rank, and, in particular, to enjoy being praised in a perfunctory, military-like style, though a touch of irreverence wouldn't hurt there either. The hard pack tells us that they are not particularly flexible in the way they deal with the world, and that could represent toughness, brittleness, or the need for protection. **Marlboro** is still the brand of the ugly American who will tend to interact with people on the basis of "this is who I am, you adapt first." If however, they choose the soft pack, this suggests a much softer side, like the America of Clinton rather than of Ronald Reagan or George Bush.

One of the men I know who smoke **Marlboro** in a soft-pack is a contractor's helper who worked around the office. His name was Jack and he followed the stereotype down to the last detail of aggressiveness: he was a working man who loved praise and macho bantering, and responded irreverently although obediently to orders. He was the kind of person who leapt at the challenge of a fight, although they tended to be of the mock sort, but otherwise, when dealing with people he was as soft and as likable as a teddy bear. The negative side? He welched on a loan from a co-worker and reacted to any discussion of this with open belligerence.

In some cases, people will develop a particularly close relationship with their brand and in certain ways the pack will assume a kind of rough correspondence to the smokers' sense of body. That means the top of the pack roughly translates to their head, or more symbolically, their mind-set. Since the top of the **Marlboro** pack is extremely angular it symbolizes the aggressiveness of the smoker. You might even describe it as prickly-headedness because male **Marlboro** smokers, like their cowboy stereotype, tend to be the kind **who** shoots first and asks questions afterwards. In my own experience I have noticed that many of these smokers have a strong, subconscious urge to seek out conflict. So, if a man you meet seems a little pushy and smokes **Marlboro**, you might as well assume that he likes to pick fights.

Male **Marlboro** smokers who seek a "safer" cigarette switch to **Marlboro Mediums,** which often suggests a slight mellowing of personality too. When a man smokes **Marlboro Lights** his relationship with the archetype will be more tenuous. The key question is whether he has moved down from regular **Marlboros,** in which case it suggests he is the tough guy open to compromise. Or, if he has migrated from another brand**,** then, depending on the brand, it might be that the smoker realizes he is not really part of the true image but feels comfortable with the diluted version. If the smoker has come from a non-macho brand like Benson & Hedges or Parliament, this could mean his macho confidence has grown, or that he is compensating for a sudden loss. Either way, he may be a johnny-come-lately, a phony, or a lightweight. A smoker who migrates from another macho brand might just have discovered his own limitations. The thing about **Marlboro Lights**, as opposed to **Marlboro Medium**, is that they have a white filter, and your best clue is in finding out whether or not the smokers are comfortable with that filter. If they are, then concealment of some kind is an issue; if they are not, then they are making an uneasy compromise. Interestingly, if the smoker chooses the **Marlboro Light** hard pack, then the chances are he will make up in rigidity what he lacks in machismo.

Among women however, the interpretation is different because they will not form the same kind of relationship with the pack. To begin with, women seem to respond to the essential slimness of the pack and this, by the way, is accentuated by the narrow typeface of the **Marlboro** logo and the "skinny legs" suggested by the "lb." That is no mistake. In the late 'fifties, Philip Morris paid Dichter $10,000 to find out if that typeface was appropriate. After much consumer research, he found that indeed it was. The effect of the typeface is a kind of visual onomatopoeia where the letters look like the image they represent, which in this case is a thin cowboy. You don't, after all, see too many fat cowboys.

Winston has never been able to speak to women, and their recent "No Bull" campaign is no exception. Their pack seems a little fleshier than **Marlboro;** perhaps the two horizontal red bands emphasize their girth. But then how could they recover from their famous first slogan, "So Firm, So Round, So Fully Packed," or for that matter, **Winston** Churchill's jowls. It will always be part of the brand's DNA.

As a result, women tend to view **Marlboro** more as an assertive or controlling force - particularly a self-controlling one - than an aggressive one. The red ribbon "roof" is perceived more as a personal control device than **as** a sign of aggression. The relative narrowness of the hard pack itself tends to work the same way.

One question left is to decide how the female **Marlboro** smoker relates to the image. Generally, women smoke **Marlboro Lights** because it feels more accessible. With regular **Marlboro** they are more likely to feel in competition with the mannish image. Sometimes women look at the **Marlboro** "roof" as a controller or a security issue, while some who smoke lights identify with **Marlboro's** equestrian image. The key issue is how people relate to their brand: do they "belong" to that brand, in which case they view the brand as a kind of psychic vitamin; or are they so far from the norm that their choice ranges from compensation to wish-fulfillment or deception of some kind.

All smoking provides some form of wish fulfillment, but smokers who "belong" to the brand are either seeking to boost their identification with the brand image or compensate for their own shortcomings. In some cases, when they seem so in synch with the image that smoking the brand seems redundant, you can consider them to be retainers, that is, people who smoke to hold on to or prolong their sense of power. For those who don't belong (e.g., a decidedly overweight, dependent woman smoking Virginia Slims) then you are dealing with world of wish-fulfillment where you can be sure the brand is offering just about everything these smokers lack. These would be compensators, and understanding the brand gives you an index of their compensation. It is important that before embarking on an interpretation that you make this key differentiation: retention vs. compensation.

Once that judgment has been made it helps to make a guess of what part of the image the smoker really identifies with. If, in the case of **Marlboro**, it is the fighter archetype, then there is going to be a certain desire to exert power. Since the characteristic is associated with the ultimately self-defeating act of smoking there is a good chance that, in the case of a woman, what may seem like assertiveness is more likely to reflect a problem with wielding power. For example, Nurse Rachet in Ken Kesey's "One Flew Over the Cuckoo's Nest" would make a good stereotype of one kind of woman **Marlboro** smoker who could only wield her power abrasively.

Marlboro Lights, on the other hand, tends to be the choice among those women with a quieter, more feminine idea of assertiveness and is usually a sign of a more integrated relationship with the stereotype. Then again, the plain-colored filter suggests a degree of personal concealment since the nipple is being disguised. Perhaps this cowgirl doesn't show all her cards?

Obviously, **Marlboro** could be smoked by a woman because she has none of the above traits; for example, a woman who is extremely overweight, not self-controlled, and lacking in any desire for power. In that case the brand is probably being chosen for pure wish fulfillment. But if you add the element of power - the desire for it or the need for it - then you are back in the realm of compensation.

Another rarer but perhaps more interesting approach is that of a woman who smokes the brand because it is related to the man in her life. One case that captures this relationship is that of a widow who begins smoking as a way of continuing the association with her late husband. The widow's assuming his old brand could become a fetish of sorts that is not an inherently unreasonable one. On one level, it certainly is a good memento but it can also go deeper. There can a be a sense of what anthropologists refer to as endo-cannibalism, that is, a kind of communion with dead relatives that, at its heart, is not at all too different from the transubstantiation ceremony in the Catholic Mass.

While as her husband is alive, a woman smoking his man's brand can also be sexy. As perfume companies have long known, the idea of a woman wearing her man's shirt or some other item of his clothing is a turn-on. But the assumption by a woman of the man's brand can also run the gamut from the essentially benign, as in the widow's case, all the way to the aggressive, as in the case of a certain military officer's wife who was in the habit of smoking her husband's brand as a way of saying "We are Captain Jones."

Finally, we can look at how brands are portrayed in movies and literature to get one more measure of how we perceive them. Granted, the placement of cigarette brands is usually paid for but, even so, this tells you something. **Marlboro** is the most common brand to show up in movies and is usually associated with soldiers and action movies. Women who smoke **Marlboros** in movies will usually be women of action. The company is famous for taking advantage of these opportunities, with the apotheosis of the **Marlboro** placement being its appearance in the Superman movie.

CHAPTER 8: INTERPRETING CIGARETTE CEREMONIES

The magic of tobacco is in the relationship smokers make with the brand. Just as each of the Balinese horse dancers act out their divine trances slightly differently, each smoker has a slightly different interpretation of their tobacco god.

The first question you ask about a smoker is, "What is the basis of their identification?" That determines whether they are attracted to a brand out of compensation or as a way of retaining, **or** holding onto, their powers. Wish fulfillment is usually recognizable because the smoker doesn't seem to have any explicable connection with a brand. If someone has no business at all smoking a he-man's brand, then, as we will see later, it could be a facade or an unfulfilled dream of some kind.

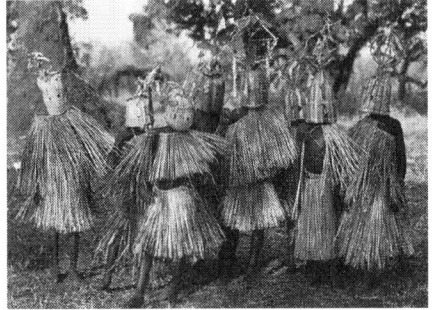

Retainers, on the other hand, seem to relate to the brand but they are smoking it because they need more - usually a lot more - of its powers or because they genuinely have that quality but not quite enough of it, or they have it and are afraid of losing it. That explains the tough-talking guy who smokes **Marlboro** to bolster his sense of machismo even though it doesn't seem that he needs to do so. What he seeks is retention. That explains, for example, the ex-marine type who obviously has the machismo but smokes because he wishes to hang on to his peak powers for as long as possible.

While most smokers are involved in a blend of retention and compensation, occasionally a person will smoke a brand that is so completely out of type that compensation as we have described it doesn't fully explain it. When that happens, it is a sure-fire signal that this person is fundamentally deceiving you or himself, or both. Thus my friend, the persistently failing entrepreneur, smokes Davidoff, the most expensive cigarettes around. He keeps his grand scheme dreams alive, no matter how unlikely. As long as he smokes these cigarettes we know he is also fundamentally deceiving himself. If he switches, then the next brand will tell us if he has awakened from his dream.

Since smoking is a personal ritual, everything about it is potentially meaningful. The brands themselves are meaningful, as is the precise variety of cigarette chosen; for example, is the cigarette light, filtered, menthol, long, and so on. But the ceremony of smoking, that is, the way in which the cigarette is consumed and the pack is disposed of, helps you shape the analysis of the smoker. The ritual tells us a good deal about the conformity, originality, or possible artifice of the smoker, since the ritual is partly self-created and partly a copy of the way his or her peers smoke, and smokers are naturally aware of the habits and brand choices of other smokers.

What are we to make of the smokers who tap their cigarettes on the pack before lighting them? If they are smoking a non-filter which today doesn't require tamping because the tobacco is well packed, this can indicate a tendency towards either useless flourishes, a ritualized hesitancy, or a desire to help or to contribute to others. The reason is that most consumers expect a product to arrive in perfect condition and don't expect to have to do anything to it in order to use it. So it is a reasonable inference that they are willing to contribute to the improvement of what should be an adequate product. This could be good or bad, depending on the situation and the manner in which it is done. If the tapping is light and subtle, it is probably good. If it is heavy-handed, it may indicate that the smoker likes to interfere with an adequate situation. If the tapping is neurotic, that is, loud and insistent or heavy handed, and particularly if this is applied to a filtered cigarette where there is no practical purpose whatsoever, then the tapping could simply be a device for calling attention to themselves.

Like most personality interpretation systems, the "tone" of someone's action is the most important part in determining what it says about that person. So does the context of his or her action. For example, if smokers tap the cigarette in the course of a conversation, they could be displaying judiciousness, as in tapping a gavel (a possibly revealing sign if this happens to be a lawyer), or trying to grab attention, if this is done in an intrusive way. If the tapping is done absent-mindedly, these smokers just might be buying time, which indicates indecisiveness or deception. If there is a degree of calculation to their tapping, such as a slow, deliberate rhythm, then you are dealing with exactly that, a calculating person.

If the lighting of the cigarette is accompanied by ceremony of any kind such as a special, often-repeated way of lighting up or the obsessive use of a particular lighting instrument, then a number of things are being revealed. Let's take a look at a few of them.

The choice of lighting instrument itself can be quite revealing. There is not much to tell from those smokers who use book matches, unless they hang on to certain kinds, like those from a particular restaurant or hotel. In that case, the source or the actual imagery of the matches is important. For example, suppose we meet someone who has a tendency to hang on to restaurant matches. Collecting these types of matches tells you that these smokers perhaps feel they are lacking in the "good life" or are not being properly fed at home. If these smokers were to hold on to hotel matches, it could mean they want to get away from things and, depending on the circumstances, this could mean getting away from home or from their existing life or that they just need a vacation. The degree of obsessiveness is what gives it away.

The choice of lighters can be a rich source of meaning because smokers are making a calculated statement with their choice. A lighter shows more of a commitment than does using a pack of matches. Often the lighter is the sign of the buff, the perfectionist, or the addict as devotee who pays homage to the "god" of smoking. People who use disposable lighters tend to show an appreciation for service and minor distinctions in life. If I were a salesman and noticed that my prospect used a lighter, I would emphasize that my product offered a service or convenience that made it a step above the other products even though it may cost more: People using disposable lighters are willing to pay for small luxuries. People using expensive lighters are willing to pay that much more but, beware, because that expensive lighter could have been a gift. So you should admire the lighter and ask its user where he or she got it before knowing exactly what to do.

The way people manage their lighters can be quite revealing because they are an expensive and entirely voluntary adjunct to smoking, performing a function which can always be accomplished at no cost with book matches. Unless they are always losing their lighters, the fact of their hanging on to them indicates a tendency to manage themselves reasonably well, or at least hold on to their possessions. Obviously, if they are doing this with an expensive lighter this tendency is even more pronounced and one can assume that these people are especially discriminating and probably quite clubbish. Or they might just be possessive.

In all cases, though, it is important to look at the way smokers set the flame and to consider whether or not the "plumbing" is exposed. When Ernest Dichter was hired to conduct a study on the popular perception of lighters, he spent some time researching the imagery associated with fire gods and the connection between fire and eroticism. Here is a description he wrote in his 1957 book, **Strategy of Desire**, on the work he did for a company that sounds very much like Zippo lighters:

"How much soul is there, for example, in a cigarette lighter? All a lighter is supposed to do is work, to do its job and light the cigarette. Yet some study of the meaning of lighters shows that there is much more to it than meets the eye. It makes fire and fire has a symbolic meaning. You create a flame. A large lighter company discovered that the sales for one model slipped when they changed the design. Why? The new design did not show the "plumbing;" it was simply good-looking, the functionality had disappeared, the inner workings of the lighter were not visible any longer. But why should this make any difference? Because a lighter, as our depth interviews with several hundred people showed, is a

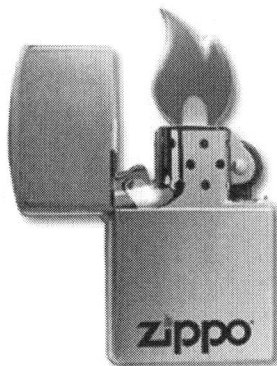

very special kind of product. You expect a lighter to work and yet you do not assume, or even desire, that your lighter would admirably perform under all circumstances. A good part of the fun would be taken out of it if this were the case. It is almost as if lovemaking were infallible. There would be little room left for masculine pride. The fact that we fail once in a while makes the perfect performance worth boasting about. Hiding the plumbing of the lighter and stressing the good looks made this model less desirable for men.

"Some readers may consider this analysis as farfetched. What proof do we have that any other kind of explanation would not serve so well? We conducted several hundred interviews, we used projective tests where people could freely associate with the designs or with real lighters of different designs. This approach then approximated a controlled experiment. Changed advertising copy produced improved sales. But even if all these facts could be rejected, another interesting storehouse of materials of an anthropological nature can be brought into play as additional evidence. As reported by Bernard Gotz, in **Archiv für Frauenkunde und Konstitutionsforschung,** Band 19, Verlag von Curt Kabitzsch, Leipzig 1933, under the title "Erotische Heilszeichen an altem Gerät," (erotic symbols on old equipment) fire-making equipment has had erotic significance in several different cultures: Lighters of a clear phallic form come from Australia and from the African grasslands of Cameroon. The Australian lighter is further characterized by the similarity of the red 'head' with the fire red of the flame."

It is amusing to think of the reaction that the cigarette lighter manufacturing executives in the early 'fifties might have had to this report. However, their marketing people, just like their counterparts in the cigarette industry, knew what to make of this. For the most part they stayed away from the sleek, concealed European style of lighters, going instead for the exposed plumbing jobs that typify American lighters. In any case, even if we are reluctant to take our cigarette lighter cues from tribal folk in Australia and the Cameroons, the association between fire and sex is just as strong in our own popular culture; we see it romantically, as in the expressions "my old flame," and "torch songs" and in the open sexuality of such songs as the Doors' "Light My Fire." That is why, even in our more refined culture, the extent of the flame is a pretty fair indication of the sexual passion of the smoker. Then again, if this is accompanied by neurosis or calculation – that is, the smoker trying in some way to draw your attention to the size of the flame - then either compensation or some kind of problem is associated with that smoker's sexual desire.

The part about the lighter concerning the exposure of the plumbing seems to work like this: Male smokers like to see parts of the gas pipes exposed while woman smokers generally don't. Any deviation from the norm is likely to say something about either sex. Exposure suggests that the women smoker is sexually open or even promiscuous, while for the male concealed plumbing can mean restraint or closeted or even deviant sexuality. Likewise, overexposure of the pipes suggests a form of exhibition in the male. When you look at the plumbing compared to the flame you can gain a sense of whether these male smokers are naturally oversexed or compensating, or whether something is distinctly out of place. In other words, a male smoker using a lighter with exposed pipes but a low flame may seem very interested in sex but may actually have a low sex drive. Concealed pipes with a high flame can tell you that something is burning deep down, and depending on other clues, that could be a pleasant discovery or an indication of sexual frustration.

Cigar smokers now use an expensive propane lighter which emits a high powered jet of blue fire. It is impervious to wind and it lights a cigar in a flash. This is an obvious power statement but also an expression of technical superiority and a way to fight frustration. How the smoker brandishes it tells the story.

The handling of cigarettes can also be very revealing. American smokers typically hold cigarettes between their index and second finger with their palm facing inward, toward the smoker. Eastern Europe smokers, in contrast, commonly hold their cigarette between their thumb and index finger with their palm facing out, away from the smoker. This is the typical way in which a cigarette is held in a French movie, whether the smoking actor is Jean-Paul Belmondo or Jean Gabin. In America, this is the sign of the rebel as smoker. For example, Bogey, the existential outsider, always held his cigarette that way and so did James Dean.

Often pseudo-smokers will give themselves away by exaggerating this pose, holding their cigarette between their first two fingers with their hand curled back too far, so as to keep the smoke away from their faces.

However, the style that Americans resent is the one where the cigarette, between puffs, remains in the extended hand of the smoker, perched between the rigidly upheld first and index finger, with the rest of the hand curved backwards and pointing towards their shoulders. This strikes us as extraordinarily regal and incorrigibly affected. It would cast the smoker into banishment in all working-class circles and most other circles, other than in some very rarefied cliques in the art world. Sharon Stone, in her famous leg-opening scene at a police station, held her cigarette in this defiant way.

We consider the cigarette between the first and second finger with the palm facing inwards the norm while the Bogey-style of "A–OK" with the cigarette between the thumb and forefinger, palm facing out, is acceptable among tough guys or people facing extreme stress. The only alternate handling style that we consider acceptable is the macho holding of the cigarette between the thumb and forefinger and with the palm out in the kind of hand signal we use to say, "it was a hundred percent." However, this is also considered overly aggressive if the smoker doesn't alternate with the more common index-and-second-finger hold or if this style is accompanied by deep inhaling. A classic example of this was General Al Haig's appearance on TV when he ran for President. He was often interviewed taking deep thumb-and-forefinger drags on a cigarette (a non-filter as best as I could tell) and the public widely considered him to be a tormented, war-mad general, and so gave him virtually no support. Overpuffing is something we see quite a lot on 60 Minutes as Mike Wallace puts the inquisitorial screws on some unsuspecting dissimulator. If this kind of smoking behavior is accompanied by collar stretching then you are dealing with someone you have caught in a lie. But if the smoker always inhales that way then he or she are probably living out a lifestyle that falsely represents their inner selves or they are profoundly neurotic.

There are numerous subtle hand formations that have many shades of possible meaning. The most common ones are the flourish and the tilted hand. These are usually the norm with women and if done with grace are indicative of some taste and artistic discrimination. In mild cases this is the same with males. However, any exaggeration denotes insincerity and, quite often, prejudice.

When the smoker's hand takes on unusual positions between puffs, this is indicative of some inner compulsion that has special meaning for each smoker. But it is definitely meaningful, usually indicating an unspoken need to deal with the world out of some inner obsession. Sometimes, for example, the smoker's hand is held above the shoulder as if ready to hurl a dart or a small sharp stone. And that's exactly what it means: this person is angry with someone or something and is looking for an appropriate target at which to aim a symbolic missile. Sometimes, the smoker's palm is held out as a sign of vulnerability; in other cases the smoker's palm may be in held in that position but in a way that seems well protected and this could be indicative of a lure or a trap. In other cases, the smokers keep their hands in front of their faces with their palms facing them and their cigarette sitting between their fingers of their hand, facing the world. This could be a shield or a mask to protect the smokers from revealing themselves. If the smoker's hand usually covers his or her mouth between puffs they are unconsciously seeking to conceal their words or thoughts. They might just be obsessively shy but you should be able to tell that from other cues. Smokers who hold their cigarette up closer to their head usually indicates that they are supercilious, as if they were saying why should I reveal my thoughts to you.

Inhalation and exhalation can be quite meaningful. Deep smoking usually indicates just that - a deep problem. But overpuffing, as we have seen, suggests panic because, as we know, when people panic, their diaphragms become tense and they cannot breath deeply. How people exhale can also tell you a lot because smokers often see their smoke as a product of their own creation. People who unconsciously well up their smoke and let it out in single bursts are saying they are able to concentrate on their work, dam it up, and focus it on a goal. If, however, that smoke is sent in your direction, then there is an antisocial quality. People who obsessively make smoke rings are either latent prodigies or, more likely, superficial enough to devote effort into meaningless tasks. As any smoker knows, it is not easy to make smoke rings and only a few can do it well. However, it is a completely useless talent and people who spend a lot of time with it are telling you just how fascinated they are with a useless pursuit.

The disposal of the pack can be revealing in a number of small ways that tell you about the smokers' feeling for the world and for themselves. The end of a pack is like the end of scene in their act of smoking. Some smokers are very uncomfortable if they don't have their next pack at the ready, while others wait until the last moment before going out for more. That message is self-explanatory. More importantly, they leave behind evidence of having smoked. The interesting thing here is that smoking is not inherently clean and smokers who dispose of their cigarettes and package perfectly cleanly are likely to be obsessive. Generally, there has to be some level of littering because the act of smoking itself is an expression of personal destruction and you would normally expect some of that to show up in **these smokers'** usage. The occasional spilling of ash, a misplaced butt, or a littered package is part of the act of smoking. So the signs to look out for are people who are overly clean, which would be symptomatic of compulsiveness, or overly sloppy, which would be indicative of anger or low self-esteem.

It is also interesting to look at the way people put out their cigarettes. If they put out their butt out in one stabbing motion you are once again looking at a sign of aggression. Sometimes this can indicate mastery if these smokers do it with grace, but it is an unhappy mastery and should be viewed as such. If a smoker takes numerous pats to get the fire out you are looking at a statement of ineffectualness - not necessarily ineptness but just a difficulty with ending something.

When smokers try to put out their cigarettes in a pile of others' butts instead of taking a clean, open ashtray for themselves, they might be telling you that they are trying to escape their own problems by casting themselves in with the detritus of the crowd. If they deliberately avoid putting out their cigarettes in fresh ashtrays, they are probably expressing an especially low sense of self-esteem, because ashtrays are meant to be dirtied. In a sense, they are saying, "I am not good enough to dirty your ashtray." If they obsessively seek out new ashtrays they are trying to "clean themselves" or rid themselves of a sense of personal distaste. If their manner is haughty it probably means they consider themselves overly important. But as long as they are insisting that you accept their dirt, there is a sadistic twist to their actions.

Another meaningful sign is the way people discard their packs. Unfortunately, there is only a 1-in-20 chance of catching smokers dispose of a pack since they have that many cigarettes to finish before getting rid of the pack. Some people have an impulse to do something to the pack before they send it into the garbage, while others can examine this last object in the trail of their smoking habits.

People normally throw their packs away pretty much as is. You may see some light crushing, which could indicate either some assertiveness or a sense of helpfulness - either informing other people that there is nothing left in the pack or providing themselves with a warning in case they think they might run into the pack again and think there are cigarettes in it. A soft pack that is scrunched up or crushed can indicate real self-anger on the part of the smoker; it may be a good idea to point that out to a smoker you love because the chances are that it means he or she is angry with themselves for smoking. A scrunched up pack probably means just that and you might want to ask the smoker what is tormenting him. Then again, you might not.

The meaning is a little more complicated when the smoker crushes a hard pack. On the one hand, it is a lot harder to do than it is with a soft pack. So when a woman crushes a hard pack it means she is an Amazon or her anger is extreme, or both. With males, it is like squeezing beer cans, except that where beer can crushing is a public expression of aggression or simply a party feat, crushing cigarette packs shows that a lot of the anger is aimed at themselves, since it represents the smoker's external image.

Smokers who damage or deface the pack in some way while they are smoking from it are displaying a sure sign they have a problem and are expressing dissatisfaction with their image or the way they relate to the world. Smokers who deface the pack when they are finished with it are displaying a more subtle sign. This common action means that they are trying to change their trail in some way, perhaps to alter what people think about them after they have gone. This action can also express regret or even a wish, perhaps, if not to quit but to destroy the evidence.

Generally, the issue for a smoker is between signaling that the pack is used up and carelessly leaving it behind. This is because all addicts instinctively know that other addicts can't resist checking an abandoned, uncrumpled pack on a table to see if their valued product is lying around. The most common way of signaling that a pack is used up is either squeezing the pack slightly or leaving the lid wide open. A discarded pack in the garbage is one thing but people who abandon their empty hard packs on tables or ashtrays without leaving a sign that they have been used up - such as slightly crushing the box or leaving it open in a way to show it was empty - might be considered as lacking in conscience or a sense of public responsibility. On the other hand, if these smokers go a great deal out of their way to leave these signs behind, then it could be that they are some kind of good Samaritan or even someone with a martyr complex.

There is a subtle difference with soft packs because it is usually self-evident when they are empty, but you never know with a hard pack. So hard packs come with an obligation to signal while soft packs do not. Still, there are smokers who somehow leave behind a soft pack that looks full; if that is no mere coincidence it means they are asking for a reaction, as if hoping someone will pick up their trail or respond to their original cry of the heart that drew them into smoking. Then again, they could be functioning in a kind of blissful unawareness or, more likely, possess a slightly arrogant sense that the world needs to accept them for what they are.

CHAPTER 9: THE CIGARETTE LANGUAGE

The Holy Grail of all studies of symbolism, from Joseph's interpretation of the Pharoah's dreams in the Bible to Freud, indicates that you need the right key to unlock the language of signs. First you need a motif; then you need to spot patterns. Today, the art of interpretation has reached a point where it is part of the language of culture from the comedy of Seinfeld to the Blonsky's semiological analysis of contemporary culture in **American Mythologies**. In the TV show Friends we find a sequence where Jennifer Anniston's sister buys a "hire-me" sweater and "rent-me-this apartment" pants. Seinfeld's specialty is taking a cultural artifact like speed-dialing and then extending it into a joke about rating a girlfriend's importance by where she appears in the speed dialing order. A simple consumer technology is now a tool for interpreting relationships. Blonsky meets with Giorgio Armani and discovers that has new, soft shouldered suit, the "sack" suit is consciously developed as a sign of the "penitent 90s." Does that help us identify the guilty rich or the unconscious losers?

Like dream interpretation, the key is to find the meaning of the dream symbol. Analysts typically do a word association test to find keyword meanings and then apply that to the rest of the dream. The art of brand interpretation is simple enough, although a few ground rules must be understood when it comes to looking at the meaning of specific brands. Much of smoking is tied up with compensation and wish fulfillment; to a lesser extent, it is also concerned with prolonging those powers the smoker already possesses. In order to read people from their brands, you must be able to make the distinction between compensation and prolongation.

Certain brands, like **Marlboro,** tie directly into a recognizable myth; in their case, **it is** the fighter/frontier tamer archetype. Because of that, while many **Marlboro** smokers are the tough frontier fighters who are smoking to retain their strength, for the most part the cigarettes are a symbol of wish-fulfillment for those who have some but not enough of the lone gunslinger qualities and a mask for others who are assuming this persona in the hopes of gaining acceptance through life.

Brands, such as Parliament or Pall Mall, that have a less well defined image tend to be much closer to the true person for the obvious reason that there is no clear "mask" value, and by being indefinable, the image, like a Rorschach inkblot, is largely being recognized at the unconscious level. In other words, it is much easier for a smoker to make a conscious statement by identifying with the cowboy in **Marlboro** since that image is quite tangible. But what do smokers consciously identify with in a more abstract brand like Merit, Vantage, or Capri? In order to make a good interpretation of the smoker's perception at the unconscious level in cases like this, it is important to have a grasp of the advertising story.

In the art of interpretation, there are unlimited permutations within each cluster of meanings. This unexpected window on the soul is filled with innumerable small paradoxes.

It is important to realize that cigarette choice always seems trivial at first, especially when you ask the smokers why they have selected such and such a brand. Superficially, their seems no different from their choice of breakfast cereal or soap powder. After all, so what? If you smoke you have to choose a brand. But why smokers choose their cigarette is different for two reasons: Smokers generally make long-term relationships with their brands, and, unlike with most other products, they are knowingly staking their lives on the practice. For that reason the brands they choose also tell us as much, if not more, about the life-or-death side of what makes them tick than any of the books they read, clothes they wear, or opinions they profess.

In some ways, digging into the mind of a smoker may seem like a dark art, since it requires a judgment on why people seek to punish themselves, but beyond that this digging is no darker than, for example, reading body language and uses much the same interpretive approach. That means looking out for compensation and reversals, and understanding context and the smoker's brand history. Beyond that, reading your smoker is a matter of informed intuition.

The structure of interpretation is relatively simple. Each brand, as it has been discussed, has a particular symbolic meaning. The smoker makes a relationship with this meaning. In cases like Camel, where the symbol largely speaks for itself, the interpretation is mostly based around the pack. With brands like **Newport** or Benson & Hedges, where the pack says relatively little, the advertising itself contains much of the message. When trying to interpret those brands, it is particularly important to have a grasp of the advertising legacy and, in some cases, the specific messages themselves.

After identifying the symbolic information of each brand, the next step is to identify the smoker's relationship with the symbolic meaning of that brand. We need to ask such questions as: Is this a form of compensation or a desire to extend or prolong its power? If it is a combination, as is often the case, what is the proportional distribution? Compensation, as we discussed, can range from having some, but not enough, of the character quality of the brand, or it can amount to assuming a false persona out of wish fulfillment. It can even be some kind of attraction to another person that has a personal association with the brand, as one might find between spouses.

Having determined the core symbolism, the next step is to consider the actual brand variation being smoked. Cigarettes are remarkable for being among the most line-extended products on the market. Virtually every brand is available in all or some of these varieties: Longs (100 mm.), hard pack and soft pack, regular and menthol, and, to a lesser extent, plain and filter.

These particular variations modify the meaning of the symbolism in much the same way modifiers work in any other language: they can enhance, soften, or sometimes transform the meaning. For example, if a **Marlboro** smoker asks for a soft pack he is telling you he has a malleable, easy-going way of dealing with people because this is against the norm; one would expect him to ask for a hard pack. Inside this smoker remains aggressive, but on the outside he makes a point of being otherwise. Depending on the person you are dealing with, this could be a softening sign on a fighting type or it could be a totally misleading sign from what amounts to a wolf in sheep's clothing. Only your judgment can tell.

The crucial part with modifiers is to know what the norm is for a brand. If as in the case of **Marlboro**, the pack is usually hard, then it is the soft pack smoker who is making an unusual statement so that this action can never be considered a neutral sign, as some signs can be. Deviations are always meaningful. You should also be aware of the norms in your own geographical area because sometimes they differ from state to state or region to region. For example, in some states such as Ohio, the norm for **Marlboro** is the soft pack and so the local who chooses the hard pack in Ohio is the one making the specific statement. The easiest way to test this is to stop by a 7-11 store or cigarette kiosk and see how the cigarettes are stacked. You can be sure they are placed in order of popularity. After all, these people sell hundreds of packs a day, so, unless they want to make life difficult for themselves, over a period of time they are obviously going to arrange the cigarettes in the order that requires the least reaching out.

If you wanted to find out how busy a store was, you could test the order of cigarette stacking against the norm, because the busier the store the more efficient the order is likely to be and the more likely it is to reflect the popularity of brands. On the other hand it, it would make you question the credibility in a scene from the film by Jonathan Demme's movie, **Something Wild**, in which Melanie Griffith and her husband, Nicholas Cage, made a practice of robbing stores by requesting for an out of the way product. While the proprietor was fumbling around for it the couple would reach into the cash register and empty its contents. The thing wrong with these scenes is that the character played by Cage is asking for a pack of **Marlboro** and the owner spends about twenty seconds fumbling around looking for it while Griffiths' husband empties out the cash register, but no storeowner would keep a top-selling brand like that in an obscure place. Either this proprietor's customers don't smoke or business is really bad. Then again, although this was Hollywood, no one thought to ask Philip Morris for product placement money. Storeowners, however, are rewarded for putting that brand at eye level.

If the brand, like **Newport**, is normally sold as a menthol, then you should pay special attention to someone who chooses a non-menthol version. The person smoking the plain version of a normally mentholated brand, e.g. **Newport** regular, is indeed an odd character, since he or she wants the illusion of pleasure without actually getting the pleasure. These options are rare enough that they are a very personal statement, and it probably means that someone, who can't stand the taste of menthols, nevertheless has a compelling personal reason to be part of the brand story anyway. As it happens, there haven't been too many brands offering this option; **Newport Red**, one unusual example, hasn't done very well. But if you run into cases like this, they are perplexing just the same. However, if the spouse of a **Newport** menthol smoker took to smoking **Newport Red**, it probably means that the couple have a sympathetic relationship.

In a reverse situation, if the brand is **Marlboro,** you should pay special attention to the smoker who chooses **Marlboro** menthols. Menthols are synonymous with pleasure and you will see that word showing up a great deal in the ads for this class of cigarettes. **Newport** ads have this built into their slogan: "Alive With Pleasure." Menthols tend to be more popular with women than with men. The interpretation of menthols tends to be a little more negative than it is with regulars because there seems to be potential for more than a usual amount of deception. But when we're looking at women menthol smokers, that should be balanced against the socialization process which tends to offer women material rewards in the place of power.

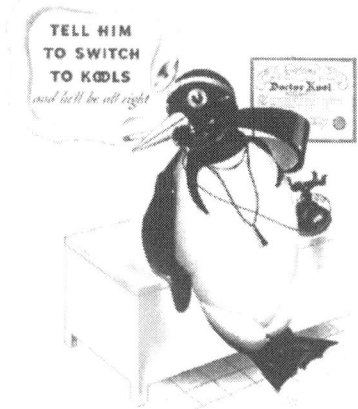

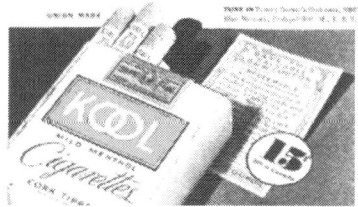

Most white male smokers find menthols cloying and believe that the menthol flavor conceals the taste of real tobacco. As a result, it is not uncommon for these smokers to say that if they want menthol they'll chew on gum and if they want to smoke, they'll smoke. So you get the basic idea that menthols symbolically stand for wanting pleasure at the cost, if necessary, of denying or masking the real thing. Very often that means the menthol smoker is a person who enjoys the elegant lifestyle over the mundane. The downside is that these smokers are more than usually susceptible to deception or, worse, will give way when it comes to a choice between pleasure and duty. Menthol smokers exist as testament to the idea that they are living the "good life."

The more substantive part of the deception is that menthols are often perceived by their smokers to be less harmful than regular tobacco. Actually, research shows that menthol smokers think their cigarettes are quite healthy, or at least, less dangerous. According to studies reported in the Institute of Medicine, "Clearing the Smoke: Assessing the Science Base for Tobacco Harm Reduction" (2001) p.78, {smokers people's perceptions of them.?} In a recent study, Hymowitz and colleagues (1995) questioned 213 adult smokers of menthol cigarettes who participated in a stop-smoking study. Among 174 African Americans, the main reasons for smoking menthols included the following: menthol cigarettes tasted better than non-menthol cigarettes (83%); they had always smoked menthol cigarettes (63%); menthol cigarettes were less harsh on the throat than non-menthol cigarettes (52%); inhalation was easier with menthol cigarettes (48%); and menthol cigarettes could be inhaled more deeply (33%). Among 39 white smokers of menthol cigarettes, reasons for their choice of menthols included the following: menthol cigarettes tasted better than non-menthol cigarettes (74%); menthol cigarettes were more soothing to the throat (51%); they had always smoked menthol cigarettes (39%); and inhalation was easier with menthol cigarettes (21%).

An industry document (Tibor Koeves Associates, 1968) reports the results of in-depth interviews (most likely conducted in 1968) of 10 African-American smokers of menthol cigarettes. The authors of the report concluded that two underlying factors "generated the great enthusiasm for menthol cigarettes." The preference for menthols seemed "based both on dynamic sensory and on psychological

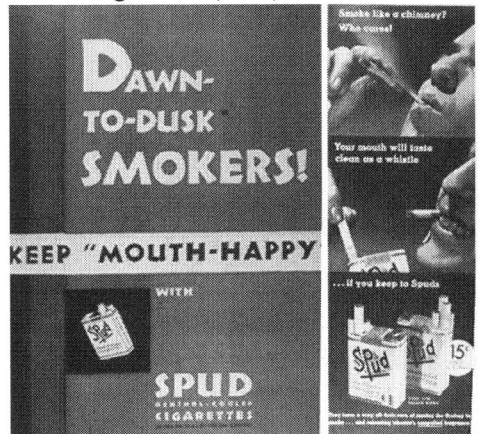

gratifications." The taste of menthol, which reminded many of candy, was a major attraction. The fact that the smoke wasn't hot or burning was also important. Psychologically, menthols were perceived to be modern and youthful. More relevant to this discussion, menthols were "considered as generally 'better for one's health.'" Most respondents viewed menthols as "less strong" than regular cigarettes, with the understanding among interviewees that cigarettes that were less strong were less dangerous to one's health.

That is why the ads almost always use outdoor settings. In the nineteen forties and fifties, menthols were actually advertised with health promises that they was less harsh on the throat. While no cigarette company would dare to make those claims today, their executives can rest assured that their customers still perceive their menthol brands as being safer. It happens to be nonsense and the smokers know it, yet menthol smokers are known to report that it feels like an anesthetic on the throat. They certainly want to believe it, so that if your menthol smoker fits that pattern, then you should know they are prime candidates for being led by the nose when it comes to issues they really want to believe in.

In general, menthols are sold with white filters. Two brands, however, have cork-colored filters: **Kool** and **Newport**. These brands have, as do menthols in general, a specific constituency among African- and Hispanic-Americans, which we will look at later. The white filter is the norm for menthols among women smokers and seems to be in keeping with the standard interpretation of deception, which can range from the mild preference for euphemism all the way to outright dissimulation. A cork filter tends to modify that, however, so the interpretation is likely to suggest that the person is more realistic or wishes to appear so. It may also be a sign of unusual aggressiveness in a woman. **Kool** and **Newport** also happen to be the menthols that most *men* will smoke, so that it is usually a flag when white filter menthols like **Salem** are smoked by a man.

In all cases, filter color modifies the meaning when it goes against the norm of cork-tipped for males and white-tipped for females. Another modifier is cigarette length. As Dichter pointed out in his Time Magazine interview, when people smoke longer cigarettes it means they want more of what is damaging them. On the other hand, length also happens to be an expression of desire. People who smoke long cigarettes, as one such brand points out, want **More**. Long cigarettes are an expression of unquenched desire or ambition. In some cases it can mean the person is insatiable. For example, I would be uncomfortable if my *banker* smoked **More**. The length could also indicate superciliousness, particularly when it shows up in brands with a special message of elegance like Benson & Hedges, but any time you are dealing with someone smoking a longer cigarette than normal, you would still have to keep an eye out for insatiability or unfilled ambition of some kind.

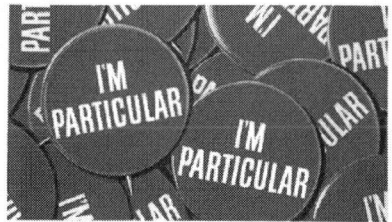

Friendly suggestion

The tar content of a cigarette is another important modifier. There is a great deal of controversy attached to this. While few medical people think that filters make cigarettes safe, they do feel it makes them a little less harmful as long as the smoker doesn't inhale deeper. And in that respect, low tars are little less harmful than high tars. No one thinks it makes much difference to the risk of cancer, but there does seem to be

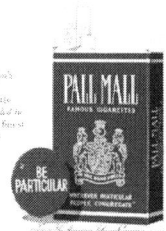

8

a reduction in less serious complaints like coughing, throat irritation, and bronchitis. Many anti-smoking people are openly skeptical, because they say these filter and low-tar devices create the impression that smoking is safe, which perpetuates the practice. That is true to some extent but, as we know, people are psychologically attached to their brands and safety per se is not the crucial issue because smokers actually desire some level of danger for "self control" purposes. Objectively, there are dozens of chemical additives like glycerin and shellac introduced to low tars. We have no idea what the effects of these additives are; they could be just as dangerous as tar. But for interpretive purposes, the only thing we need to pay attention to in the low tars is the relative frequency of smoking. If people use low tars to be healthier but then either smoke more or smoke more deeply, they are deluding themselves and that should also be considered as a general character statement.

In general, high tars and non-filters express intensity, so whatever the symbolism might ordinarily suggest, it now becomes heightened. If the smoker is "prolonging" machismo, then their fear of losing power is that much more intense and potentially that much more troubled; i.e., there is a deep fear of fouling up. In this day and age, however, the image of non-filtered cigarettes is so negative that it actually reflects a kind of desperation. It could be the brand of an outlaw, an extremist, someone who really hates him or herself, or a person who considers himself a "real heavy." Mike Wallace, of 60 Minutes, for instance, used to smoke Pall Malls – a long cigarette without a filter. If you were going to be interviewed by someone on TV bearing a long cigarette, which indicates dissatisfaction or unfulfilled yearning, and the self-destructive intensity of a non-filter, its overripe red package is your warning: its logos are traditional but its intentions are largely destructive.

There are additional symbolic meanings to the Pall Mall brand, but Mike Wallace's look of unhappy intensity is perfectly reflected in his choice of cigarette type. One interesting point, however, is that Pall Malls were originally advertised in the nineteen fifties as being safer because they were longer. Their amazing claim was that since the smoke had to travel further the extra tobacco length cleaned it. A Pall Mall smoker is likely to believe that increasing the scale may justify an otherwise unsavory act, a point that many of Wallace's ambushed TV subjects may agree with.

A not very common signifier is the color

Pall Mall's natural mildness is so good to your taste!

of the cigarette. Most are white. Occasionally a brand shows up in the color brown, such as **More** or **Sherman**'s; the latter is the product of a well-known New York tobacconist. The color brown is especially associated with power but when the choice is, for example, Sherman's, then power is often indicated in a shabby, indirect way because these cigarettes are really compromised cigars. Since cigars are supposed to be the proclivity of rich old men such as bankers and robber barons, a brand like **More**, which is both long and cigar-colored, is, in effect, a feminized cigar so a strong message of power and ambition is being expressed. If smokers choose the more fashionably-colored light brown **More**, the message is more integrated with femininity, but the basic meaning remains: When men smoke these brown cigarettes they are likely to be phonies. The reason is that their cigarettes are skinny and they don't give an "honest" smoke that is the full-bodied flavor of a cigar, so are considered by men to be there just for show. The male smoker either knows that and smokes them anyway - a sad picture - or they're unaware of it, in which case he is exhibiting many of the above negatives, plus the additional one of being a socially myopic.

The final modifier is the pack itself, which we have already discussed. The pack tends to relate to the way the person expresses him or herself to the outside world. The norm is the soft pack, which reflects informality and pragmatism. The hard pack is indicative of rigidity, fanaticism, concealment, or the need for protection. In terms of distinguishing the symbols and the smokers' interpretation of them, it is also helpful to think of the top of the pack as relating to their heads, the middle to their bodies, and the bottom to their feet. The pack can also relate in a loose way to the id, ego, and superego and in some brands specific messages are made at each of those specific levels.

For smokers, having knowledge of their practice does not in itself get them to stop smoking. The real benefit of this knowledge is that it teaches smokers the mysterious pull their cigarette brand has over them. Then, if they wish to quit, they will know what psychological compensation or repositioning they are going to need once they do give up smoking. The fact is, nothing replaces smoking, so if people do give it up, they need to know how to deal with the unfulfilled psychological needs that tied them to smoking in the first place. Smoking after all, did not solve those needs, and they can quite readily deal with them in other ways. But first they must know what they are, and their choice of brands can help identify them.

Knowledge of brands also gives smokers special insight into what makes them and other smokers tick. For non-smokers, this knowledge illuminates an age-old mystery that also provides insights into culture and the fundamental dilemmas of living: the battle between the sexes, between the generations, and within one's self. If you are a smoker and have a mind to quit or love someone who does, the knowledge of brands may be a cultural wave with which to ride out of the habit.

SECTION 2
Inner Quitting:
How to Get Beyond the World of Cigarettes

A Really Intelligent Way to Quit

There are really two parts to quitting: the physical part and the mental part. As the Science study of heavy smokers who quit after damaging their *insulas* shows, the mind approach is a much more powerful route to quitting than is the physical approach. In fact, smoking is arguably all about a mental charge that smokers are getting from their brands. That might explain why many successful quitters say something like "I just decided one day and I quit." That would sound maddening to the smoker who, like Mark Twain, feels that quitting is easy, "I've done it hundreds of times!" But it shows that being psychologically ready is far more powerful than any patch, gum or medication you can take. There is no harm in using these aids, of course but the real quitting is within.

The purpose of this book is to help split the two battles apart and fight each one separately and on their own terms. Neither Hitler nor Napoleon could fight a war on two fronts, so why would you succeed? First you fight the mental battle and then, when you are ready, the physical battle. You don't want to be at war with icy Russia and sunny England at the same time!

In fact, this is the technique I used to quit when I began writing this book in the nineteen eighties. It is not necessarily the quickest way and it may requite more honestly, insight, and research than most stop-smoking methods. But once you quit this way there is just no going back because you are taking out all the magic that smoking has for you. Once smoking has no magic for you, there is simply no reason to smoke.

The key to this technique is *unsmoking.* By that I mean you roll back your years to the time you didn't smoke and retrace the steps that led you to smoking. This is where a basic understanding of the brand meanings is critical: They help you understand what cigarettes meant to you, your friends, and your family at the time you began smoking. Then you factor in the coming-of-age process and the way in which it bonded you to the smoking habit. You need to develop a transition process, whether it means you replace cigarettes with healthier practices or simply move on.

Often too, there is a deeper ceremonial side to smoking - something with a near-religious sense. In that case you will have to develop a ceremonial way to put the old bond to rest and create a path to a liberated way of life.

The cigarette brands are rich with meaning; you can gather this from understanding the key idea of the brand as well as its story over the years. Typically, successful brands wind up fulfilling a need in the marketplace even if they didn't quite start out that way. That need explains why a brand like **Kool** can appeal to blue collar whites as well urban blacks or why high society **Newport** became the preferred brand for urban Hispanics. The mother of all tobacco transition tales is **Marlboro,** which helps explain its appeal to young white males, cowboy wannabes and various constituencies of women.

How Smoking Still Gets People – How They Can Get Out of It

Since the $25 billion tobacco settlement there have been many changes in the world of smoking. For one thing, the climate of acceptance has disappeared, and smokers have become the pariahs of the new millennium. But the reality of the settlement is also that government at every level is deeply dependent on the cigarette taxes and the payout bounty. Only a tiny portion – overall, about 5% of the billions paid out each year - go**es** toward the youth tobacco issue.

At the same time, it is clear that even though the cigarette demons costs more than double the old prices, the demon has not been slaughtered. Perhaps this is the critical moment when the parties will be interested in the more substantial underlying issues of tobacco and perhaps of all vices.

The most significant advantage of this knowledge, however, is for personal use. When I began developing the underlying theory of cigarette language and ceremonies and showcasing them in conferences like the Popular Culture Association convention and in articles in Newsday, US News, and other publications, the concern was always that the tobacco companies would be the leading beneficiary of these ides. However, over time it became clear that smokers themselves are the ultimate beneficiaries because smokers possessing fully detailed knowledge of their relationship with their brands is the true key to permanently quitting.

As these chapters describe, committed smokers – that is, addicts who adopted smoking during their teen years - have developed an identity bond and mythic-level attachment to their brand. Many smokers are either unaware of this or have simply forgotten what smoking meant to them when they started. Yet, in order to quit they need to resolve the issues that got them started, renegotiate the deal with the vice, and then seal it at a meaningfully ceremonial level.

This is hardly the condition-response method traditionally employed in most quitting techniques. But that is not to say that it replaces them. You may still need those techniques. The point is that if you do not resolve smoking at the psychic level, these techniques cannot work, so you wind up repeating what Mark Twain once said: "quitting is easy, I've done it hundreds of times." This technique addresses the issue of motivation, most everything else address the surface issues of practice.

CHAPTER 10: THE MEANING OF THE MAJOR BRANDS

Traveling through the Berkshire Hills, we come upon a strange new phenomenon: a series of anti smoking billboards. They look hip, youthful and, though a tad hard to read, they tell us a seemingly critical piece of information: "**Marlboro** dominates the under 19 marketplace."

Thousands of dollars have gone into telling people the obvious: most young white males smoke **Marlboro**. Unfortunately, not one penny has been spent on telling them why. If these young white male smokers knew why they smoked this brand, there might be something we could do about it. Indeed, the same can be said for all the ads in the Truth Campaign, which paint the tobacco companies as villains. They probably are. For that matter, so are the commercials, which are effective with many teens. But that only applies to teens who really don't need to smoke, not to the ones who are at risk for smoking because of personal reasons. And it does nothing to help the committed smokers.

The simple story about smoking is that it delivers the Hero myth to youth. Smoking fills exactly the role that anthropologists have always seen in initiation rituals in strange, primitive cultures. Yet, what very few have been able to fathom is that the myth is being delivered to us – to our kids – in a consumer product with an image cultivated from much psychological and market research.

It would be entirely fair and accurate to say that **Marlboro** has in effect hijacked the American Hero myth and sold it as an addictive product. **Marlboro** has in effect become the standard Hero myth because there are precious few alternatives to a youth who wants to experience the thrill of taking the forbidden journey in the hope of coming back with the prize.

A lot of urges go into smoking: power, sex, status, and personal control myths. Cigarettes also provide a psychological gratification that can ameliorate the typical teen neuroses, with issues of self-esteem, self-control, and sexual urges being high on the list.

At a congressional hearing, a teenager was once asked why she smoked. She said that she saw a TV psychologist talk about cigarettes being used by teenagers with depression. Since she was feeling depressed at the time, she thought, "Hey, that's what I should do."

The Chthonic Urge

What stumps so many who deal with the teen smoking issue is the power of teens' urge to try this or any other forbidden element. The mythic urge to find one's role and begin the journey – or rather to find one's mission - is chthonic, that is, it comes from the earth and there is no stopping it. It is every parent's nightmare – the runaway urge, the runaway quest.

That very force that drives teens is part of our regenerating life power but it may also be our downfall. If we deny it, we choke our power to regenerate, but if we let it go its own way it becomes the destructive killer force of nature. And sometimes we just can't do anything about it.

In that light, let us take a look at the handful of brands with which teens begin their life's smoking journey. This is what makes them stand on frozen sidewalks in the middle of winter to grab a quick office puff. This is what consigns them to the sad community of other smokers' company as they stand together, sending a haunted, resentful, and ultimately defiant glance at the passersby who wonder, "Why on earth would they keep doing it?"

Marlboro, the key white male brand followed by the distant second, **Winston**, is a metaphor for the Hero experience. Teens want to be challenged, so the test is whether they can endure the smoke of this product. The payoff is the association with the American Frontier Warrior myth and a modern age medallion package as reward. The offer is simple and well supported with a billion-dollar ad campaign and association with key sporting events of a dangerous kind. There is also a huge merchandising business associated with collecting **Marlboro Miles** – that is, smoker units – that can be redeemed for the kind of stylish outdoors items and smoking paraphernalia that a good cowboy might naturally carry. The **Marlboro** initiation memory is so broad that it could almost be meaningless, except that it inherently relates to conformity. The **Marlboro** teen is less the modern-day pioneer than he is a youth asking to be regimented. If you can figure out these **Marlboro** teens' "fighting association," that is, which warrior concept they adhere to, then you can understand what they are willing to organize around. When we add the greater contextual information - their peers and parents' brands and their alternate and taboo brands - you get a much better picture of their inner needs.

When girls initiate with **Marlboro**s they are making a statement that they wish to either challenge or be made available to the lead warrior class, to become the local alpha male. Or they may be defining a complex pas de deux with the male principle in their lives.

In either sex, when the martial or for that matter conformity urge is slightly lower than the norm, they will initiate with **Marlboro** lights. But **Marlboro** lights are in a soft pack that uses gold, while regular **Marlboro** are in a hard pack with red-blooded coloring. So the statement and the kind of psychological satisfaction are different: Less passionate, perhaps less committed, and less rigid.

Nowadays, you can also go with **Marlboro** Milds, which have the advantage of the **Marlboro** traditional look and feel, but without the personal damage. Its message is something akin a marine who figures out how to get an office job.

The girls still think you're tough but you're not spending as much time in harm's way. Unfortunately, it does say Mild in big letters so you assuredly lose face among the alpha-male seekers. Men too, are making a similar compromise. But for those comfortable without that level of pressure the brand represent a reasonable compromise.

IMAGE ANALYSIS OF THE MAJOR BRANDS

WINSTON

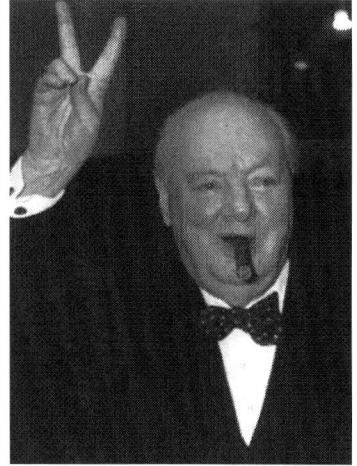

Winston is the leading brand for talkative males and a minority of wanton females. It was the first macho filtered cigarette that preceded **Marlboro** in the early nineteen fifties. It was the product of RJ Reynolds' headquarters town of **Winston-Salem** but it was also coincidentally blessed by the postwar afterglow of Britain's heroic smoker – and talker – **Winston** Churchill. Its ads were macho but not focused as **Marlboro** was, on a single character. Its key selling point was its poor grammar, as in: "**Winston** tastes good like a cigarette should." This poor grammar thus scored points with intellectual rebels and lowlifes alike. The spirit survives today in the brand's association with NASCAR. Its occasional lascivious ads attracted certain blue collar women and those women who wish to signal overfamiliarity with men.

In the nineteen fifties and sixties, **Winston** was the leading filter tip brand for adults but at the end of the sixties it gave way to **Marlboro**. Without a central image, the brand lapsed and, according to internal documents from RJR, it suffered because their choice of ad characters, who seemed to follow traditional pursuits like golf and helicopter piloting, became associated with the unpopular and losing Vietnam War. **Marlboro**'s image grew in part because of the decades-long mythologization of the West in film, but also because the passing of the frontier in real life and the civilization – read feminization of the frontier male – has added a great deal of nostalgia to the brand. The brand has achieved what myths of Jason and the Golden fleece, the M'swati myth of the Basutos, Camelot and the Merlin Myth,

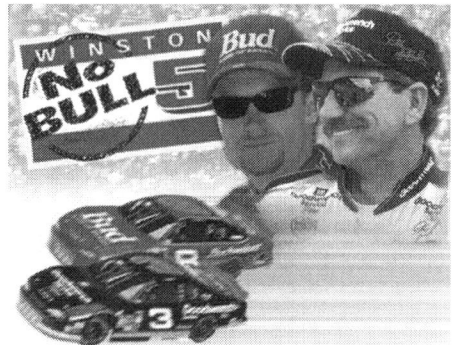

and even Harry Potter have: chthonic force, that is, the eternal power of ideas coming up from the earth's core.

People look to this brand as a metaphor for their life force and, as they get older, as a lifeline to their passing youth. Fortunately, we can now say that with the right strategies you can take control of the psychological implications of your brand.

A white male who initiates with **Winston** signifies a more gregarious person who has a macho association with mechanical objects. This gregarious aspect is derived from the source of **Winston**, that is, its historic association with **Winston** Churchill and its "king size" crown on the pack.

Today, that image has been altered by the brand's association with auto racing. The **Winston** cup has helped cobble the brand under this new banner and this association will stick in the minds of many.

In the past few years RJ Reynolds has appeared to pre-empt the health issue with **Winston** by declaring there are no additives in the tobacco, which is an obvious lie since it is impossible to make cigarettes today without some additives, and also by going for a "Natural" and "No Bull" statement in their advertising. "No Bull" is the one that seems to have stuck. It has the secondary appeal for the gregarious smoker - the classic talkative **Winston** smoker - who is reassured by smoking this brand that his blather is truthful.

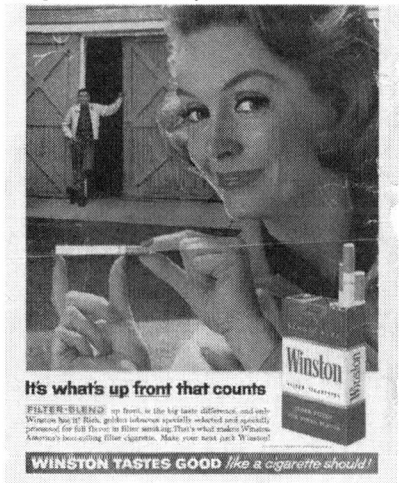

It's what's up front that counts

WINSTON TASTES GOOD *like a cigarette should!*

When a woman smokes it, the brand takes on a different meaning: it suggests a tomboy but more likely a woman who is particularly interested in the company of many men, if not sexually, then certainly with high degree of familiarity.

CAMEL

Someone at RJ Reynolds may have been thinking zoos, but the public has been more interested in sex, particularly that of the base, hairy kind. At one point **Camel** was a man's thing but in recent years the brand has appealed to a certain kind of woman interested in the flamboyant display of animal magnetism and has culminated in a new version of the brand called Camel No. 9.

Camel is the first great created brand, in contrast to brands such as Lucky Strike, which seemed to appear out of nowhere or that occurred out of chance or whimsy. Here the RJ Reynolds Company had the benefit of experience, a known selling concept, and some early twentieth century research.

When it was introduced in 1917, Camel was intended to be a good ol' American brand that would compete with those pesky Turkish and Turkish-style cigarettes that were sweeping the marketplace. The top brand back then was Murad but there were also many others with Turkish or even Egyptian symbolism. Back then the Middle East was perceived as an exotic place and the true home of great tobacco.

Camel was conceived as an American brand that would harness the oriental imagery, use a smidgen of Turkish tobacco – so they could say "Turkish & Domestic Tobaccos" – and gain market domination. From the point of view of tobacco technology, Reynolds was taking advantage of developments that enabled them to take cheap American tobacco and give it a Turkish flavor. American cigarettes with Virginia tobacco, a newer, cheaper white burley, which lacked flavor, was introduced to replace American cigarettes made from Virginia tobacco, which was once great but also expensive. The advantage with white burley is that it is extremely adaptable – a kind of blank page of tobacco that could be made to assume virtually any flavor with a series of additives that included things like sugar and cocoa. Nowadays, that list of additives has grown to include such terrifying substances as glycerin and ammonia, plus a host of additives that sound like the contents of a chemical waste site. Smokers are increasingly more likely to be inhaling the insides of their cleaning closets than actual down-home tobacco. (Hence **Winston**'s No-Bull and American Spirit's "purity" appeals).

Camel also had the advantage of a quietly popular brand to model itself on called Red Kamel. Oddly, this brand has been revived today as a special, "chic" version of Camel in an attempt to appeal to the smoking aficionado – the person they suspect could be lost to American Spirit or premium imports.

Where the Original Red Kamel featured an Arab on a runaway red camel, the idea was to slow it down and get a stationary shot of Joe the Dromedary against the backdrop of some distant pyramids. We'll never know why, and at what subconscious level, the early twentieth century Reynolds executives saw a penis. But we really don't have to know, because at some level this image appeared to strike the right note. We know now, both by the obvious phallic references in the notorious Joe Camel cartoon images of the nineteen nineties and by a process of elimination, what the camel actually stands for. Back in the 'seventies, in an effort to modernize the Camel, Reynolds essentially gave the Camel a haircut and removed the warm exotic background from the pack. Sales drooped.

Like Classic Coke, the original brand was returned to its place of prominence. Only this time, the manufacturers understood the association, and within a matter of years Joe the Cartoon Camel with the extremely phallic mouth made the point clear. The brand is about sex and the package says penis. We can also thank a small French ad agency for identifying Camel's essence and developing this character.

The initiating male, it may safely be assumed, is being drawn by matters sexual and may as easily be compensating for sexual needs as seeking to assert some kind of control. If a female initiates with this brand, she has clear issues with the male organ, which could range from simple sexual needs to dealing with issues of personal abuse, or to displaying mannishness in a lesbian or implied lesbian context.

The Camel ad campaign that followed the departure of Cartoon Joe has consistently worked on the appeal of Camel to attract women – and to women it has sold itself with a deeply sultry image, in essence, a really tough slut. It is as if a woman were wrapping herself around the male symbol to push out her femininity. She could have a weak or missing father issue, or she could be competing with men as much as attracting them. For men, this may seem like the ultimate turn on – like a woman wearing nothing but your shirt - but in reality she could actually be trying to punish males. In other words, she could just be trouble.

VIRGINIA SLIMS: "THE GREAT LIBERATING BRAND"

Virginia Slims is the brand of the liberated lady, or so it says. In fact, the brand is a feminist tease: a trapped, mousey woman wishing she were tough, or a harridan hoping to add some allure to her ways, or any number of possibilities in between. It is to the feminism what American cheese is to *brie*, not the real thing, not very healthy but for many people, the best they can do.

Feminists with backbone need not apply!

The cigarettes themselves are long and skinny like great legs and the name Virginia, with its virginal association, is probably the least liberated of women's names. Likewise, its famous ad campaign, "You've Come a Long Way, Baby," is hardly the phrasing likely to win over the heart of a Betty Friedan. Then there is the issue of a dry, reddish coloration on the pack which looks oh so much like dried blood, thereby suggestion that this brands empowers the smoker with a sense of control over her love-hate relationship with menstruation.

Supposedly, while **Marlboro** is King, Virginia Slims is Queen. She shares that title with **Marlboro** because so many women also smoke **Marlboro**. This is probably of no great concern to Philip Morris, since they own both brands. But we obviously care a lot because Virginia Slims has done a great job of evangelizing smoking to the only domestic growth segment left: women.

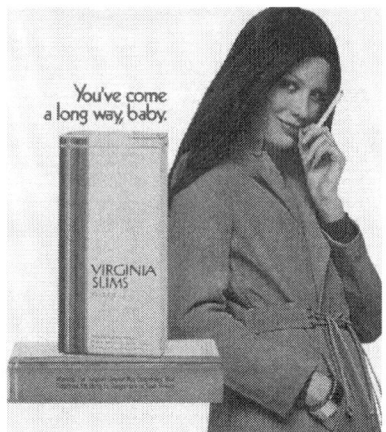

Virginia Slims Tennis Is Slammed Again

The amazing thing about the **Virginia Slims** brand is that its entire strategy was already mapped out in 1922 when Edward Bernays – Freud's American relative - made his client, American Tobacco, put Lucky Strike on the couch. The psychology was simple and the analysis of Freud's American disciple A.A Brill crackles with all the force of pop psychology: "The cigarette has become the modern woman's torch of freedom."

Clearly, the same people who hijacked the American Frontier Hero myth had very little trouble recognizing the American Liberated Woman myth and went to work so much more self-consciously. The research had already been done by the consultants hired by psychoanalysts in the twenties. Women may see cigarettes as a torch of freedom but in order to be useful they also need to keep women slim. Hence the earlier "Reach for a Lucky Instead of a Sweet" commercial for Luckies by George Washington Hill, which was not a brand statement but rather simply a potent observation about cigarettes for women that had previously worked for Luckies. Virginia Slims later co-opted, so before there was a Virginia Slims there was a famous campaign that established cigarettes as a dieting device. Virginia Slims was now adding a political statement to the promise to become or maintain slimness.

Finally, the brand has to reflect the girl's passage to adulthood, which is her journey from virginity to nubility. Hence the name: Virginia Slims.

The cigarettes are also a few millimeters slimmer, thus creating the physical illusion that the cigarettes do the job of slimming. Then the ad campaigns haul out the mock history of women's hard-won right to smoke. The net effect is true brand building in the form of myth imitation. The brand is now real and its clever comic approach has effectively hijacked the liberation myth. It is as if Lucy

Gaston, the suffragist, anti-smoker, and unsuccessful Presidential candidate, was reinserted into the history books as the first great woman smoker. This was, of course, a huge irony when you consider that she ran on the cigarette prohibition platform.

It is also no coincidence that the brand package bears a more than passing resemblance to dried blood, the transition period of menarche or simply the sense of control over menstruation.

When we put this all together we have the portrait of the brand – its magic and its edge. This brand offers it all: a promise of slimming and a subliminal suggestion of controlling your body. The smokers of course, would have to be a bundle of contradictions and misgivings to want this brand but that is a good description of a teenage girl. Is it a surprise then, that a majority of young white teenage girls initiate with Virginia Slims? It is saying all of the right things, despite all the right warnings on the pack.

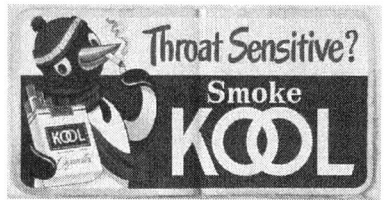

KOOL: PSYCHIC LIGHTENER FOR AFRICAN AMERICAN SMOKERS

The **number** 1 selling brand among black Americans is Kool. In general, menthols are favored (according to the study citing RJ Reynolds' own figures in Washington Post, January 15, 1998; p.1 par. 15) by 89% of African-Americans in contrast to 27% of whites. There really is no creation myth for this brand or for this phenomenon. In its early days, Kool was associated with iciness and, not too indirectly, good health. The first menthols, such as Spud, promised to be easier on the smoker's throat. This brand was meant for smokers who were literally burning out on regular cigarettes and either wanted to "smoke all day" or needed a taste of candy.

Kool was once the choice of caucasian blue collar workers. But somewhere along the way the brand was discovered by black Americans. Today menthols are standard among African American smokers, and Kool has become a brand that likes to use ads with jazz horn **Players** (breath power, naturally) to associate itself with a kind of Miles Davis, a rebellious, strangely mysterious figure, where the warrior image is more the slick inner city *Shaft* than the cowboy of *Shane*. And yes, they are "cool."

hen there is a following among white lower class stereotypically "trailer-home" clientele. The ads focusing on this

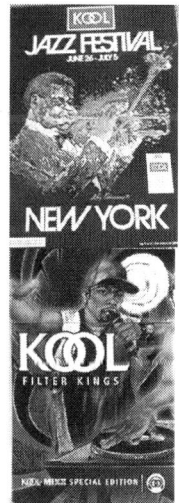

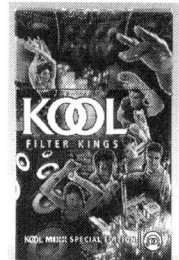

group don't say much, although the message is roughly the same but very differently interpreted. There is another class of white people who are attracted to black culture as the transitional pack on the left shows. However, for their traditional clientele they, like most menthols, have had to abandon the 'fifties health claims in cigarettes. So Menthols use the association with a number of things to make the health point: the outdoors, skiing, snowcapped peaks, cigarettes that look too clean and pure to be unhealthy, and a number of unlikely images that represent the smokers' idea of everlasting pleasure.

The knock-off menthol brands such as Philip Morris' Alpine and even the menthol line extensions of regular brands use the color green to indicate the

pine and ice suggested by the product. But to African-Americans the flavor really represents a way of adjusting to a white world – by becoming "whiter" than white, by being "kooler."

To black people, menthols first appeared to be a brand that offered the psychic equivalent of a skin lightening cream and a simple pleasure dividend in a society that made them feel less than comfortable. Now, menthols have become almost entirely co-opted by the African American community and it is simply the norm. It is, in effect, the black **Marlboro**.

SALEM MENTHOLS

The alternate brand to KOOL is **Salem**. It has a much smaller following and is more common among women. It is also the menthol that whites, especially white women, will smoke. The brand tries to look slender and has recently undertaken a makeover from its simple green stripes on a white background to darker green on lighter green with a new yin-yang type of logo.

Like Camel, this is an old brand whose identity was only truly understood long after it had been established in the public mind. To R.J. Reynolds, **Salem** is just the other half of their hometown's name, **Winston-Salem**. It was their filtered menthol offering of 1954. To smokers, however, that is another story.

Salem, like **Marlboro**, has a history that most

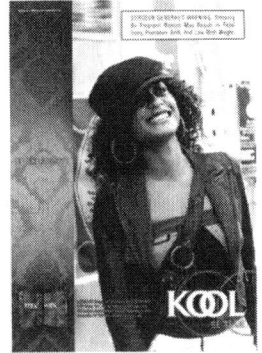

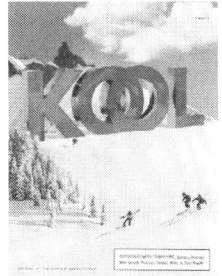

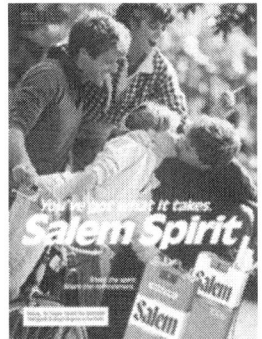

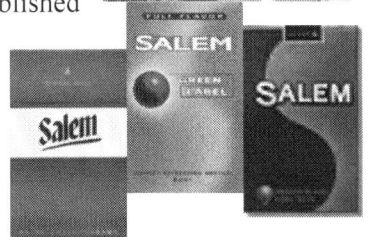

people know something about. While it is true that **Winston**'s association with Churchill is fading and therefore remains as a kind of vestigial brand residue woven into the DNA of the product, **Salem**'s associations remain still very much alive in the minds of any American. While few may be aware of the specifics of the Pilgrims' witch trials, the name **Salem** remains synonymous with witchcraft and the supernatural. Therefore it is natural to assume that people, especially women, see smoking this brand as a way to express, or compensate for, their sense of inner spirit power. This smoker may be the beloved the muumu-wearing earth mother, or the pushy realtor who sways you toward the three bedroom, one bath Cape Cod house in a dubious neighborhood because she has the exclusive brokers' listing.

Generally speaking, the Pilgrim history was less relevant to the black community, which tended to see this product as a more feminine version of KOOL. But, over time, R.J. Reynolds must have found that its spirit association was a great enough power that it could be exploited in a world of tattoos and body piercing. So the brand moved toward a kind of universal spirit power with the redesign of the pack and the introduction of a new ad campaign aimed at the tattoo set, called **Salem** Spirit. In this new incarnation, the brand is represented a kind of green yin-yang symbol and oriental snake-dragon that looks like good tattoo parlor material.

In a swift move, the product has made itself relevant to a young, body-conscious, pseudo spirit- seeking market. It will likely become a viable alternative initiation brand for the teen non-conformist, especially attractive to the odd-ball artist wannabe, the narcissistic biker, the anti-cheerleader, the follower of any pseudo-cult from a heavy metal lover to a biker who values pleasure.

It is worth noting that **Salem**'s redesign has caught up with the original contention of the original Cigarette Seduction analysis of the brand, that it was related to "spirit power." In the beginning, the analysis of **Salem**'s underlying iconology was simply not reflected in their very bland advertising campaign. In the nineteen seventies and eighties and even into the 'nineties **Salem** ads did little more than show their name against snowy mountaintops with fresh pines. Occasionally, the ads tried to glamorize their smokers with a Cosmopolitan look showing independent but sensual women. But as the Cigarette Seduction analysis made clear when it was first introduced as the "Cigarette Semiotics" paper at the 1984 Popular Culture Association Convention in Toronto, successful initiation brands have to be about more than good looks - there is always a powerfully iconic event below the surface with deep cultural resonance. In effect, this is a brand that survived and even flourished, in spite of its poor advertising. Eventually, when a new generation of marketers finally put this brand on the couch, they

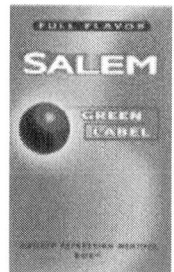

discovered what the Cigarette Seduction study had maintained for over a decade: a brand associated with the first, albeit tragic, act of female power in this country would hardly remain unnoticed among a population seeking "spirit-power" from their tobacco habit. We sort of congratulate RJ Reynolds to catching up to our analysis.

NEWPORT

This brand, which manages to attract an unusual coalition of adherents, is within the same range as the menthol pleasure seekers. **Newport**, sporting its abstract sail package and its obvious association with old wealth, is a symbol of the upwardly mobile and the leisurely rich. However, Hispanics are the growth segment for this brand; it is the brand of choice among the East Coast's primarily Puerto Rican community. Generally more attractive to males than female, **Newport** is also a choice among both male and female whites who share the sense of easy striving.

Like Kool, **Newport** can be described as a male brand because it has the key ingredient of a male brand: the cork colored "nipple" filter. **Salem**, on the other hand, remains the choice of women because it has the white "bra" colored filter.

Newport, however, bears a peculiar advertising history because it did its research early and identified its key references back in the nineteen eighties. It has been the subject of a highly controversial but effective ad campaign. To begin with, it got its message dead on: "Alive with Pleasure." What more could you say about a menthol? The pleasure principle reigns supreme while the "health" benefit is front and center.

However, all smoking research will reveal a dark side. That dark side is part of the reason people smoke. It is normal to find anger, self-blame, loathing, and a kind of free-floating death wish among smokers. Typically, these impulses are incorporated into the campaigns through the background or through incidental ways; for example, the **Marlboro** Man is not the picture of health but rather is a grizzled, hardy man who is a product of his dangerous environment. In other examples, **Winston** has always tried to associate itself with risk-taking activities from auto-racing to helicopter flying and Camel has gone after mountain climbers.

According to the campaign analysis made by US News columnist, John Leo, in a Spy Magazine article in 1987, the highly visible **Newport** couples ads – the ones showing men and women having fun together - were fraught with domestic

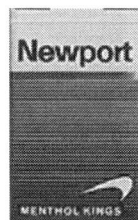

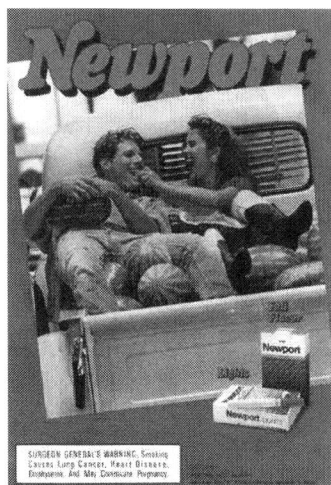

violence and sexual imagery. In Leo's highly revealing analysis these apparently fun-loving ads were shown to be stagings of symbolic acts of fellatio, wife-strangling, husband-beating, and simulated violence. The ads would show the man playfully holding his hands around the neck of his woman companion – a symbolic act of strangling? A woman would be shown drinking out of his spurting hose – as if it were fellatio – and, in another ad, playfully aiming some violent object at his groin.

As a true journalist, Mr. Leo even contacted the photographer who took many of these shots. Not only did he deny any knowledge of what Mr. Leo was talking about, but he was shocked, shocked to hear of such accusations. What *was* Mr. Leo thinking?

The photographer may indeed be telling the truth because the shots were conceived by the ad agency and the manufacturer. They evolved out of the larger vision of an ad campaign and the images were already sketched out by the agency's art director long before the photographer arrived on the scene. It is quite possible that, once he got into the swing of things, he added his own seemingly innocent ideas. But the fun and sadism-below-the-surface is understandable when you consider the real messages contained within a product that inherently deals damage to its users.

The question is, what does this say about domestic violence? While the **Newport** campaign has become much more tame over the years, it remains part of the brand DNA and it is still an issue. Is this brand the stereotype of the wife beater, or, for that matter, the husband beater? It certainly could reflect the choice of one **Newport** smoker I know who embodied the calm, joy-loving person on the outside who was a diligent owner of an enterprise while suffering a long marriage with an alcoholic wife. To him, the brand was a summation of his station in life and deathly reward as well. While each smoker has a unique experience, it is likely that this experience will encompass some elements of the campaign. It is the rare smoker who consumes a brand in spite of its image.

MATURE BRANDS

The brands in the next tier are rarely used as initiation brands; rather, smokers tend to migrate to them. When teenagers *do* initiate with these brands they are making a strong statement; they are either trying to skip a stage in development or overly identifying with an adult. Teens in the thrall of Svengali would smoke their brand and an outsider might choose one of these brands to display superiority.

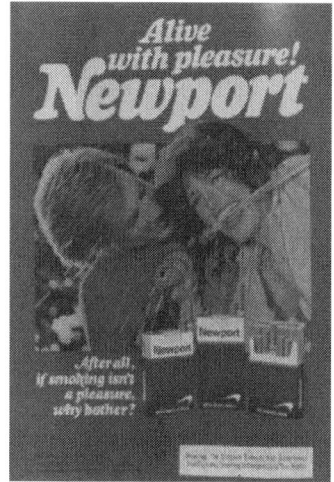

KENT

This brand, with its English castle – its Connecticut Yankee in the Court of King Arthur sensibility – makes it the choice of the patrician, whitebread smoker. It is also the choice of the wannabe, the society acceptance-seeker person on the path toward upward mobility. For two other reasons, it is also the choice of the concealer and dissembler.

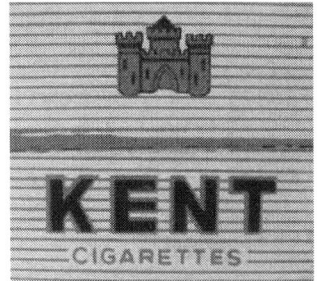

Kent has a white filter tip. While that is the norm for women it is not the norm for men, and so a man smoking **Kent** – which *is* the norm – is inherently about concealing something, whether it is a simple personal restraint or downright concealment. Inside the filter is something else: the great charcoal-activated micronite filter. At the scientific level there is some evidence that these tiny chunks of charcoal do indeed clean out the smoke to some extent. The final effect, for the average smoker is less "taste" and more "purified" smoke, but that is subjective. On a symbolic level, however, the charcoal filter is something else: it is about whitewashing dirt but with other dirt. It is therefore not unreasonable to look at this smoker as someone will save face at all costs.

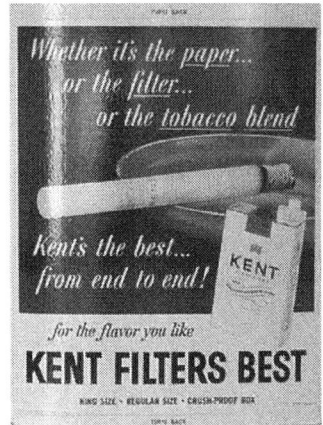

These charcoal-activated filters are especially popular in both Japan and the United States. **Kent** is a very popular brand among Chinese and Koreans, who perhaps saw the international TV campaigns of the early nineteen sixties, or perhaps the castle actually looks more like the Great Wall. It may be that the concept of the micronite filter "refining smoke" symbolizes industriousness; perhaps the upward mobility of the image speaks to their drive

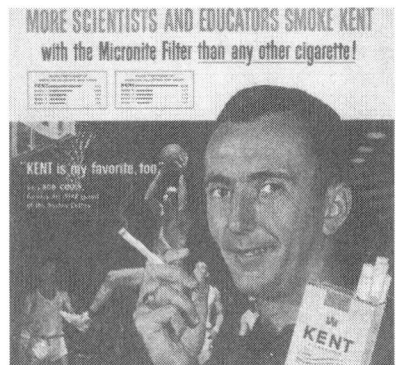

for work and entrepreneurial success. Generally speaking, however, **Kent**'s ads don't say very much, but if they ever adopt new ads you can be pretty sure they will go after their unique hybrid of WASPs and Asian strivers.

CARLTON

With its promise of 1mg of tar, this has long been the brand of wannabe quitters. It is also the brand of health-conscious starters, that is, the kind who only want to be a little pregnant or the person who believes that drinking a little of the poison that is already hurting them may even help. It is symbolism – in this context – tends toward the unfortunate. It has the abstract symbol of an Indian, but not the sturdy, totem-like the cigar store Indian who represented noble conquest; rather, this is more like the head on the tombstone of the unknown soldier-Indian - the lost people and the lost soul who identify with this guilt are the kind who grieves for them but can't really take the last step to change, to alter the past, to make something of it. Finally, **Carlton** can be the brand of the quitter who just couldn't do it, the brand choice of the tenuous and also the victim, the guilt-seeker, even the martyr.

It is important to remember that if a smoker is actually quitting, then this brand, as a waystation to cessation, is just fine. But as an actual brand choice it stands for all of the nebulous qualities discussed above. Overall, as a cigarette, it may also be the mildest coping stick available, and for that we are sympathetic. However, most research seems to indicate that low-tars are generally ineffective because people seek out a certain level of nicotine and will puff harder at low-tars to get to the nicotine level they are seeking, which means they bring more destructive smoke into their lungs, thereby offsetting the lower tars so that the net result could be more unhealthy. So the real issue in judging Carlton smokers, or the user of any other extremely low-tar product, is: how hard do they draw? If they draw hard, they are fooling themselves. If they draw light, they are genuinely highly tempted to quit. It is then a question of whether they stay that way or move on to healthier things.

AMERICAN SPIRIT

This is the smoker who throws himself to nature, magic, and history rather than face up to the reality of **his or her** addiction. In younger people **this** is a creative, sensitive solution. In middle age smokers **this** represents surrender to a habit they cannot quit. So some degree of guilt or self-loathing or transmutation of guilt into hip pride is inherent to the brand.

You could even argue that American Spirit is *kimo sabe* to Carlton, its spirit brother and possibly true partner. Where the Carlton smoker is likely to be uptight and uptown, **the** Spirit **smoker** is all downtown and loose. Hey, why go with the abstract, phony, dead Indian thing when you can inhale the righteous, original thing. Here we see the inherent self-deception of smoking move to a new level. The core promise of the brand is hey, this is what the Indians did and look how close they were to nature. So if it was good enough for them, why not for you? In smoking this brand, the smoker has the option of feeling at one with the historical source of this land, a sense of making up for the past sins of the white settlers or a kind of rationale that says it can't be bad if it was a critical part of native culture. Some people will even imagine that by smoking this brand they may be helping the Indians.

Clearly, the meaning of this brand is different if you are indeed a Native American smoker but for the vast majority of its customers none of this is true. So the issue in looking at American Spirit smokers is to determine which of these elements these smokers most strongly adhere to, and then you will understand their manner of wish-fulfillment: Are they a "brave?" Are they hiding behind history? Are they expressing self-loathing, going native, or simply rebelling against the West?

BENSON & HEDGES

While rarely a teen initiation brand, it may work as a sign of gayness in a young male except for the occasional queen bee teen hoping to exude an air of exclusivity. After all, it is based on a distinguished British Brand, – and it comes with its own little royal crest, or coat-of-arms, and a glittery pack. In adults, it is also a popular choice within the gay community.

While the brand now stands for a kind of generic class superiority – obviously born out by its extra length, 100mm size, its brand history has quite a different dimension.

When **Benson & Hedges** was launched in the nineteen sixties by Wells, Rich & Green, a hot new ad agency co-founded by Mary Wells, a kind of Mary Tyler Moore prototype in the ad world, the brand became famous for its TV commercials. These poked fun at this cigarette brand's extra length by showing scenes of the cigarette being bent or cut off in the course of ordinary working situations. So a worker on a ladder might find the cigarette hitting a wall and its extra length would bend. Or a window shopper would find it hitting the window and then bending. The emblematic ad was the one in which the brand got caught in the guillotine-like closing of an elevator door. In other words, the American Benson and Hedges is a brand which deals with castration, or in its abstract form, it

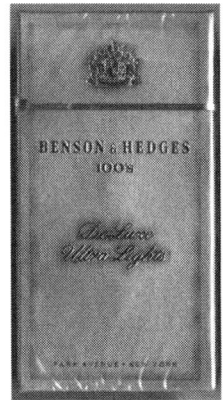

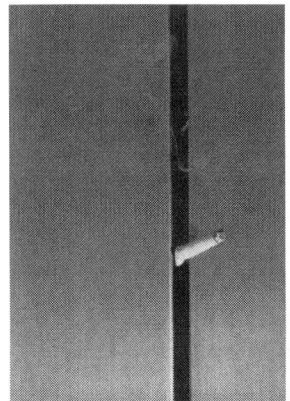

ranges from emasculation to a sense of cutting someone down to size. Or, it can reflect the more complex personality of a self-aggrandizer who somehow undermines him or herself.

Generally, this is a brand people will migrate to at a later stage in their smoking career but, in any case, in the process, this brand reflects an interest in elevating one's status and a possible willingness to do it at another person's expense. It can also be symptomatic of the deeper issue of cutting down to size or a conflict with self-elevation or defeatism to the point of self-mutilation.

LUCKY STRIKE

This brand is now long past its prime but it hangs on and is occasionally dusted off and staged for a revival which never seems to work. Anytime there is a 'fifties revival, Lucky Strike gets a little shot in the arm because it was often the brand teens wrapped under their T-shirt sleeve. It was originally a brand of loose tobacco that dates back to the nineteenth century gold rush days. The brand appeals to the risk-takers who hope to hit the big one, such as a gambler or a hell-raiser, but also at one time the majority of American smokers from 1920-1950. It was the smoke of choice when America really struck it big in the early twentieth century; it stayed with them when they almost went broke in the depression and stuck around with them during World War II. It was also the most relentlessly marketed brand of its time, thanks to George Washington Hill, the prototypical advertising huckster. It eventually changed its pack from green to white, during war**time** after long realizing that the green had to go. Since copper, a minor ingredient in the green ink, was a strategic wartime product, the change was supposedly done in the national interest with the campaign slogan, "Lucky Strike Goes to War." Opportunism runs deep with this brand but sadly, all for naught, because the white Luckies spelled the beginning of the end for the brand.

Luckies also thrived with the once famous but now forgotten slogan in the nineteen forties and 'fifties, "Lucky Strike Means Fine Tobacco," which is a mnemonic that survives on their package as L.S.M.F.T. But this is all in the past. Once George Washington Hill wasn't around to push the brand anymore it went into a natural decline. When it is smoked now it makes a specific reference to the past and has little current significance.

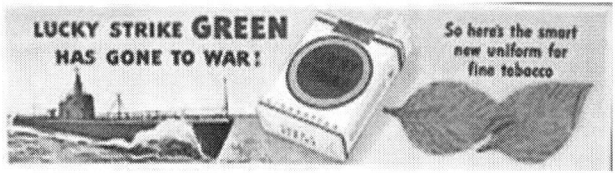

PARLIAMENT

This is a brand without a clear image, so smokers tend to bring more of their own baggage to this one than to most others. You can assume that smokers who love the two shades of blue and a chevron are somewhere between slightly depressed and bi-polar and also crave recognition. This is a brand for smokers who set themselves apart from their culture, but without leaving the United States or buying a foreign brand. The strange "recessed"

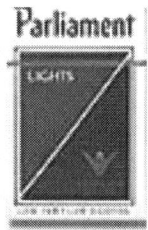

hard filter suggests these smokers have issues with communicating that may include a need to vent or sharpen the old tongue.

Digging into the soul of this brand shows some interesting aspects. Parliament ads often show couples and the ads used to reference England (Parliament, right). in ads. When that lost its cool, a smart person in the marketing department noted that democracy comes from Greece, which also has these exotic islands, so that ought to be the source of our modern day Parliament.

Rarely is this an initiation brand. On the other hand, it is an unusual cigarette because of its strange stiff plastic filter. Since the smoker is seeking the reassurance of the nipple, this plastic-covered item suggests a coldly unloved or unloving side, or perhaps even cold calculation or cold pragmatism. Since the filter is recessed - in other words, the mouth doesn't make contact with the actual filter - there is a suggestion of hiding or disconnecting, or more likely a need to disconnect, from the true volume of one's statement. The mouthpiece may be the chewy, ruminative cigarette holder a la FDR or a kind of microphone for stentorian announcements. It

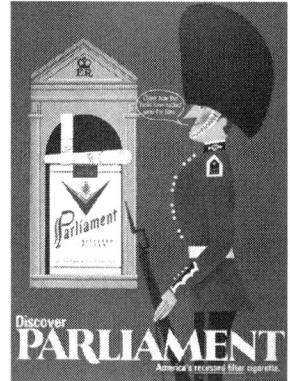

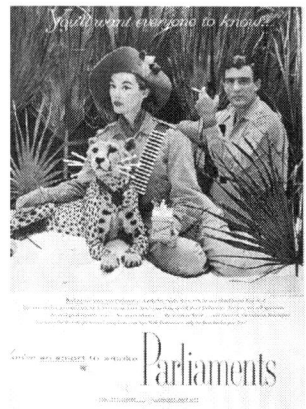

is obviously not a macho brand and its democratic message can suggest diplomacy or argumentativeness. It could often be the sign of a judgmental personality, but not necessarily the quiet type.

The twin blue colors on the pack may also suggest mediation of a diplomatic sort or transition from one lifestyle to another, or from one world to another. Since parliament is a foreign institution, usually European, it is way for the American smoker to claim an out-of-the normal identity. This might not be as much European as just a statement saying, "but not quite among the rest of us."

It not often an initiation brand, but when it is, it is a sign of aloofness or an affectation of superiority or just "apartness." It is also a great brand for the passive resistant personality.

DECLINING BRANDS: MERIT, VANTAGE, EVE, TARRYTON....

BARCLAY

Since this is the brand that coincided with this author's early research – by creating a kind of urbane hero – its miserable failure is viewed here with a peculiar mixture of glee and sorrow. Launched in the early 'eighties with a $125 million campaign, the idea was to create a James Bond-like image. My research showed there was on opening for an urban hero with a gangster-like scar, a kind of spiffy mobster. While the obvious image was an urbane sort of gangster image in a white tux, Brown & Williamson's eventual campaign had gone all James Bond; instead of the scarface (a scarification ritual that Africans often use for tribal branding in lieu of tattooing) their face had the much tamer cleft chin. The old chin dimple not only took the danger out of the brand but also created a barrier, since this is a genetic gift – not something a tough person can earn on the street.

The greater problem is that the James Bond thing is just not American enough to be true myth material, so the product floundered. Oddly, my research anticipated the appeal of John Gotti, the "Dapper Don" who turned out to be a very appealing rogue. Since none of these occurrences are connected, the brand now occupies a space that says low rent English-cad-wannabe. Good luck, and, might I say, good riddance

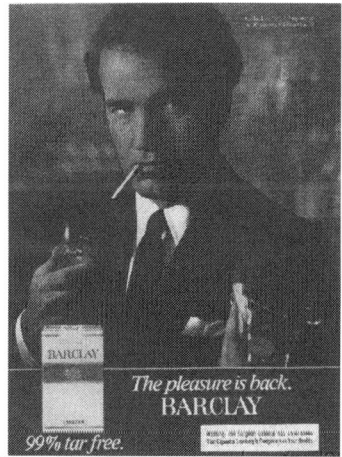

MERIT

There was a period when Merit had some…..merit. That was when the middle class still smoked, at least in a way where they were still comfortable doing so in public. At that point – and this would be in the 'seventies – when the cancer scare widened into the emphysema, heart failure, and other bodily damage scares, tobacco companies needed to counter the image nightmare scare by developing brands that let smokers save face as they lowered the carcinogens. That was **Merit**. The symbolism on the pack spoke towards "going forward, go on with life." It also resembled a chart – a stock or a medical chart – and so it seemed both scientific and rewarding.

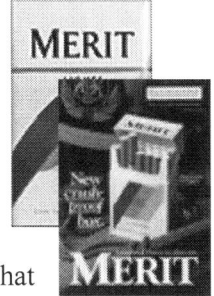

Interestingly it also resembled the graphological view of the universe, which puts the tops of letters (the l's & h stems, for example) into the superego, the middle zones (m's & n's) in the ego zone and the lower portions (the y & g stems) in the id. In the case of Merit, the strongest coloration remains in the ordinary ego zone. Not too smart and not too sexy.

Upper Zone: Mental, Intellectual & Spiritual
Middle Zone: Everyday and Social Interactions
Lower Zone: Instinctual & Unconscious Drives

So, contrary to its name, there was little emphasis in the superego or intelligence portion, thereby indicating little Merit after all. In reality, you can't use intelligence to sell tobacco, as Rosser Reeves discovered back in the nineteen fifties when he used the slogan, "When you think about it – Viceroy," to sell the first filtered smoke in the wake of the early cancer scare of the late 'forties. The obvious reason is that if you think about it – really think about it – you wouldn't smoke at all.

Since tobacco is neither rational nor intelligent it makes no sense to appeal to the rational mind. As a result, Philip Morris does very little to promote **Merit** and most of its low tar smokers have moved on to **Marlboro** lights or some other brand like **Parliament**, where the suffering personality rather than the sexual side is addressed.

VANTAGE

Reynolds' contribution to the smart smoker stakes was this brand, which had a peculiar filter with an inverted cone of empty space within. Why they thought that a filter with less filtering material in it would do a better job, is of course a great mystery. Nevertheless, the brand

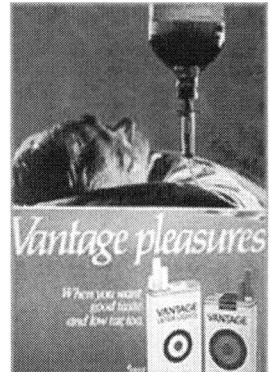

did attempt to appeal to the public's metaphysical sensibility, such as the Vantage Point (one of its headlines). But the ads often used cords and lifelines; the most obvious was the oxygen lines and a deep-water suit on one of their ad layouts. The implication was of course that it offered an umbilical chord and that the smokers existed somewhere between wanting their connection restored to their Mommies or the age-old examination of one's belly button. Fortunately, the brand is in deep decline and we are no longer required to solve this riddle.

THE OLD BRANDS:
PALL MALL, L&M'S, CHESTERFIELD, OLD GOLD

Few people smoke these brands today and they are rarely advertised. In the case of aging smokers, their references simply date back to the golden days of those brands. These few surviving smokers can be dated and even understood by considering the images they conjure up when they are smoking those brands. It is a way of preserving their younger days. Younger smokers who pick up these brands are making somewhat deliberate references to these old days.

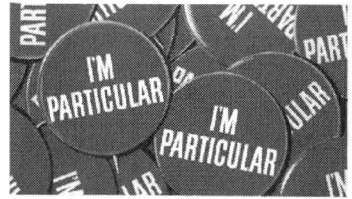

Friendly suggestion

PALL MALL

Pall Mall is still a working brand. It was the choice of smokEnders founder Jacquelyn Rogers and 60 Minutes anchor Mike Wallace before they both quit. It's an older person's brand – the color of an overripe tomato – and seems to reflect a certain weariness with life, a kind of been-there done-that cynicism. That old pain is reflected in the name, both because it has old British connotations (Pall Mall is famously wealthy section of London) and because of its association with death – as in "Pall" (like pallbearer) or even self-destruction, as in "Maul."

The historic absurdity of this brand is that it was once advertised as being so long that the extra tobacco acts as a kind of filter. Its common form is unfiltered so it is definitely the choice of the tough or truly self-destructive – read depressed – smoker.

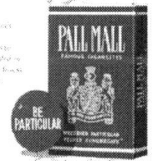

Pall Mall's natural mildness is so good to your taste!

When a young person takes on this brand he or she is expressing a range of messages, from wanting to be older and sager before their time to also willing to be more destructive. The index is that of self-destruction, which is a general rule of all smoking, but is especially apparent in a long cigarette without a filter: just how far down to the butt smokers can smoke. Too little and they are dabblers, too much, and they in a troublesome mode.

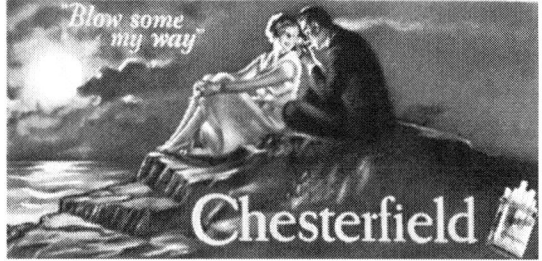

CHESTERFIELD
Chesterfield is rarely seen these days but over the past 20 years or so, there have been some mild attempts to mount a comeback. It is a nostalgia brand with a sense of the Old Country Club set. There may well be some WASPY types who will reach out to this brand as a gesture of retro longing. However, today this would translate into something more like a field of chests, – i.e., a graveyard – and only someone with a twisted sense of history or morbidity would smoke it.

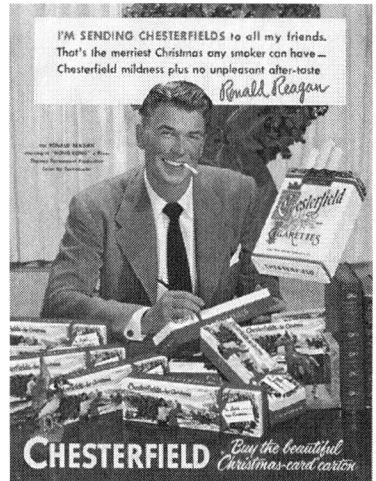

OLD GOLD
Old Gold is remembered for its dancing girl cigarette packs of the nineteen fifties and the infamous slogan: "Not a Cough In A Carload." The simple explanation for anyone still smoking this brand is today is – a loser. Let's face it, there is no gold, new or old. But there are also more charitable interpretations: someone who pines for a lost time or is hanging on to a legacy of the past, someone with something in their mind that it is evocative of "old – and probably tarnished - gold."

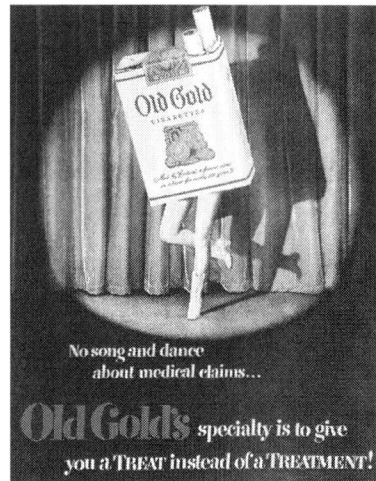

"TRIBUTE" BRANDS
As the price of tobacco rose and the negative

publicity began to undermine society's once open acceptance of smoking, cheaper brands arose. Initially, they were no-name brands that appealed to mature smokers who just wanted to save a few cents. As cigarette prices rose dramatically and public disapproval grew, the issue of saving money teamed up with a sense of "Who cares what brand I smoke." Now, the price of smoking has reached the point where it is acceptable to smoke a decent looking no-name brand. Even younger smokers will occasionally intermingle their critical initiation brand with a knock-off, sometimes feeding in them into their **Marlboro** packs in order to keep the image alive.

Few of these brands have achieved any kind of imagery of their own that warrants examination. The way they are analyzed is simply by finding out what brand the smoker migrated from or intersperses with their cheapo brand and then do some type of math based on the cheapness and inherent lack of authenticity.

However, some derivative brands have achieved an authentic, if modest, brand value in their own right. **Basic**, **Buck**, **USA** and **GPC** are some of the bigger ones.

Basic says just that and in many ways is the precursor to the No Bull ad campaign that **Winston** uses. This is the Puritan workman brand, the lowly wage slave, the salt of the earth or the person who fancies himself as a kind of scout. These smokers would be as close to being good honest citizens who are thrifty and without too many illusions about giving up on their old habit. The negative side is likely to be a desire to cover up a difficult or more complicated situation or to recover from that situation. This is a good brand for a fellow going though a divorce or a bankruptcy.

Buck would be the woodsman idea of **Marlboro** on the cheap. Huntin', fishin', and drivin' a mud-splattered pickup truck and drinking lotsa beer come to mind with this brand. It is a country person's identity tag. It would be especially meaningful if **it were** smoked in the city but passé in the country, where you would associate it with a pick-up, gun rack and a strung-up deer in the yard.

GPC is the brand that Homer Simpson or a blue-collar stickler might go for. The idea of a brand as an acronym tends to appeal to the blue collar shop steward, sports coaches, and corporate middle management boosters who love insider codes, mysterious abstractions, and mnemonics. It makes smoking sound like a mandated practice and therefore coldly acceptable.

USA: Wrapping yourself in the flag has a way of making a bad habit feel a little better. It may be low-rent patriotism but it does tell you something vaguely sincere is there or perhaps it just masks something insincere......

READING THE SMOKER'S PERSONAL MYTHOLOGY

It would be a dull person indeed who wouldn't attempt to put all the brand information together and try to get a read on the individual smoker in his or her acquaintance. After all, we look for meaning in people's choice of such things as their car, clothing, and favorite TV shows. With cigarettes however, the meaning reaches deeper because it is always associated with this initial passage in people's teen years and so it defines their key flaws and their personal vision quest. It also defines what they are willing to sacrifice themselves for. Smokers will always attempt to trivialize these matters for the obvious reason that they have no interest in putting such personal information on display. But they do it anyway by the act of attaching themselves to public brands that share a kind of collective meaning.

The challenge is to find out how each smoker personalizes that meaning, especially since they may be projecting one level of meaning while identifying with another. In other words, we have to determine the level of compensation while trying to understand what they are giving allegiance to.

Smokers give clues; for example, often they move on from their original brands due to life changes or crises. Most smokers are willing to substitute one or more brands if they cannot get their brand of choice. These are clues too. So are the brands they *will not* substitute for.

In the end, what we are looking for is a system of self control and image projection. It tells us what the smokers wish to control or even punish in themselves and what they want the world to think about them. So there is the outer brand – the tough cowboy exterior of say, the **Marlboro** smoker which makes the ego look good – and the inner brand which is there to feed the id. For argument's sake, an urban bookworm who wants to compensate for the years in which he felt bullied may choose **Marlboro** for the way it makes him pass for tough on the outside while on the inside this brand remedies his inner sense of weakness. Or he could be tough guy on the outside who bolsters his sense of inner toughness because he is not sure he is tough enough or he fears losing his tough edge.

The difference between the two is the way smokers handle the habit: the tough guy tends to deal with the cigarette naturally, while the compensator is likely to reveal some unnecessary ceremony in the way he goes about smoking, such as perhaps even acting overly macho.

To get a better read, we want to know the smoker's satellite of substitute brands. The history of the brands he smoked may provide some idea of why he couldn't stick up for himself or what general set of weaknesses and yearnings he or she has. Most of all, we have to understand how it started. What, if anything, did the smoker smoke? What did he start with or what did she first bond with.?

Interpretation is the one great art that everyone takes a crack at. At some point in the process the genius looks about as good as the fool. And there are people – clairvoyants being high on the list – who don't even seem to go through a process; they just appear to know. The difference is in understanding the key elements that resolve the uncertainties. In the world of semiotics the term for interpretation is "hermeneutics." It can be great fun to read academic tomes about the art because they are themselves, generally uninterpretable.

The art of interpretation is simple enough in concept but turns quickly complex as the number of relevant sign options increase. The true art of interpretation is in finding the key element that resolves all the mysteries. In technical terms it is about "disambiguation," that is, which element resolves most of the ambiguities. In this approach, interpreters generally look for one or a series of standout features, develop a hypothesis, and then check to see if all the elements are resolved by it.

Cigarette brands, like any other symbol system, have ranges of meanings which combine differently, depending on the key principles. A type of grammar is employed, and these elements, while not absolutely irrefutable, are usually quite constant. So the three issues of filter type, cigarette length, and packaging are relatively unchanging and can help the interpreter make sense of the smoker. The brand history and smoking style (e.g., heavy draw or puff-puff, disposal of the cigarette or the package) also holds a depth of meaning.

The greatest clue is always going to come from deviations from the norm, and frequently that is the disambiguation factor to look for. For example, a weasely man who cracks the filters off his **Marlboro**'s is telling you all about compensation. Remember, he could always buy a non-filter but chooses to tamper with or destroy a regular brand. His general smoking manner, and how hard he draws, can tell you if he is angry or simply yearning or if his pain is lingering or sharp and of recent occurrence.

Deviations from the norm are always the best place to start because they are most glaring and most initially revealing. But they are also somewhat treacherous because they can also mask complexities, so be warned. For instance, if a man smokes a woman's brand he is not necessarily a homosexual, although that would be a reasonably good bet; **he** may be working for a woman and using this brand as a way to express submission at one end but also anger at the other.

We are much more accepting of women assuming men's roles, so a woman smoking a man's brand is not necessarily a major flag, except when the brands have adopted a "primitive" male role. Greasy mechanics and smelly cigar smokers are typically the exclusive realm of males who tend to relish foulness as a natural barrier to female intrusion. Therefore, when a woman assumes that role it is inherently an aggressive statement. Depending on the context, that statement could range from extreme man-hunger to a yearning to appease the memory of a father to a direct challenge to the male role, if not his authority per se. Or it could be a type of fairly heavy-handed seduction such as those suggested by the occasional Camel for women ads.

Disambiguate accordingly!

Smoking a brand deemed acceptable by a particular group is a time-honored way to gain entry into that group. As smokers feel more embattled by legislation and smoking restrictions, the more they are likely to appreciate a new member to their camp. On the other hand, the group may also be alert to a phony, so the brand better fit the person according to the way the group see things – or else.

When people of color smoke standard, non-menthol American brands they are making a statement. The most likely statement is that are adapting to the so-called mainstream; presumably, although not necessarily, the white mainstream. But that would be the statement. If an African-American spent a lot of time with whites he might adopt **Marlboro** as his brand, or he might gravitate in shades from Kool to **Newport** or **Salem** and then either to a standard brand or to the menthol version of a standard brand.

The reverse is true of a white person who spends a lot of time with African Americans. He or she might adopt a menthol, perhaps moving from a menthol variation of his standard brand to **Salem** and at the moment of most acceptance or most denial, Kool itself. It is not unusual to find a white jazz musician who plays in an integrated band smoking menthols.

Since the historic association of menthols is with ice and cooling it is not uncommon to hear of white people who have suffered burn trauma pick up a menthol.

There are also smokers – of all races – who, upon feeling burned out on smoking have moved to menthols. It doesn't usually work and of course smoking menthols has no health advantages, but that is part of the illusion of menthols.

When it comes to understanding people who adhere to the norm, the issue is always tougher because you don't know where to look. If a tough cowboy or a beefy cop actually smokes **Marlboro**, and no doubt many of them do, then the obvious question is, what are they compensating for? Older smokers may fear that they are being perceived as "over the hill" in their job so they smoke **Marlboro**. Adopting a new brand is a sure giveaway and the nature of the smokers' fear is quickly revealed.

In a more complex situation, you would look for more subtle clues that are less obvious deviations from the norm. A tough guy who moves to **Marlboro** lights or even **Marlboro Milds** could be slowing down or, in his mind's eye, becoming more mature.

Another key is when a smoker violates the cigarette grammar: men are supposed to smoke cork tips, the ones with the nipples; women, generally are not. Most smokers want a soft pack, except in the case of **Marlboro**. Here, the norm is the hard pack, their outer personality, which suggests that the smoker has a tendency to be harder, more brittle, and more defensive, as if he or she is hiding something or, if the smoker is using a soft pack, suggests a softer, more flexible attitude. A smoker who likes a brand, but is uncomfortable with the norm, may chose a variation such as a soft pack **Marlboro** or a menthol variation.

If someone moves from a long cigarette to a shorter cigarette it probably means they are becoming a little more realistic in life, that they are giving up their grand obsession. Or it may be a sign that they are becoming a little more health conscious. Dichter was once quoted as saying that smokers who go for longer cigarettes are just playing Russian roulette with eight chambers instead of six. Actually, that would lower their odds of dying, so that should really be about using two bullets instead of one! But that does raise the issue: do smokers think it is safer to smoke a longer cigarette or do they just want more out of smoking?

Generally, extra long cigarettes indicate unfulfilled yearning or ambition and the issue of whether smokers see it as safety or satiation is an indicator or their personal rationalization. In other words, do these smokers yearn for more in life or are they just getting a better bang for their buck?

Age Deviations

When older people either cling to the brands of their youth or suddenly adopt a youth brand, we know they are acting because fear of aging. It may be a sign of mid-life crisis if a man who has been smoking **Kent** or even **Winston** suddenly switches to Camel. Likewise, a woman who has been content with Doral, a budget brand that has a modicum of pseudo-brand appeal, switches to Virginia Slim, is signaling her yearning for a return to youth.

When teens adopt an adult brand, that often means they are trying to become mature, rather than older. That sounds almost good except that it is fundamentally false and is usually a sign that they are imitating the behavior of an older person they admire or whom they associate with the brand. It is very important to establish who that person is since it could signal an inappropriate relationship.

Complexity

The art of brand interpretation takes a big step forward when we get to learn about the constellation of a smoker's brands. What will that person smoke if the store is sold out of their his or her brand? What will that smoker accept if offered a smoke at a party and what brands will he or she avoid, preferring to have a nicotine fit rather than have a smoke?

Granted, it is not always easy to discover this but it is worth asking. This information always disambiguates. A **Marlboro** smoker who will take the occasional **Winston** is a little gregarious. If he refuses one it may well mean that he despises talkers, yackers, and salesman. He might even be downright antisocial. If a smoker is willing to take menthols, then it is a sign he wishes for an easier life. If he or she would rather die than smoke a menthol, this suggests that person may be a little judgmental. Generally, the alternate brand information helps us disambiguate.

The most accurate reading, however, comes from a smoker's brand history. If we can know every brand that a person has smoked, we will know the journey of his or her psyche. This includes every brand that smoker experimented with – and when – and then every brand he or she has used as a substitute. The key here is to determine which brand he or she has made a conscious effort to go out to acquire because every time they do that, they are responding to the message contained either in the advertising, or, more likely, in the packaging itself. This reflects a psychological need.

This is why, when people are in crisis or somehow in flux, they may switch brands or do strange things with their existing brands. They may tear off the filter, thereby indicating that they need a stronger dose or are feeling more self-destructive, or they may move to the stronger or weaker variation of their existing brand.

The smoking ceremonies can often be revealing, especially when they deviate from the norm. Unusual holding that either reveals or conceals the smoker's face can be meaningful. Careless disposal usually means that the smoker is angry or defiant. The way in which a smoker extinguishes his or her cigarette can be revealing. Are they putting it out in one sure push, which shows a form of decisiveness? Or are they putting it out with an indecisive series of pitty-patty dabs? Do they make an issue of stomping on the extinguished cigarette? Do they try to conceal the cigarette, perhaps under the sand or under other people's butts, thereby demonstrating shame or lack of self-importance?

Package disposal plays a role too. Most smokers will do a kind of rudimentary, almost ritual checking of the pack to see if anything is left before they toss it into the disposal. Are these smokers poor, stingy, or just very careful people who will check thoroughly to see if anything remains. If they don't, these smokers could be careless or just feeling wealthy. If they crush the pack – an obvious sign of anger – the question becomes who are they angry with? Are they angry with themselves or the world at large? Or both?

When smokers try to actively disfigure the pack, such as tearing the box or ripping up the package, then something is eating at them. Sometimes there is a pattern to their disfigurement: they could be attacking their own self image or they could be unconsciously isolating the element on the pack that has special meaning for them, in a sense, reaching for their personal talisman

SOME SAMPLE INTERPRETATIONS

A teenage smoker starts fitfully at first with **Marlboro**. Let's say he comes from a blue collar background. Let's say neither parent smokes. So, in a way he is breaking new ground. Perhaps his starting to smoke shows conflict or distress or maybe it is just a break with the past. He goes to community college but at some point sees a shot at getting into a state college on a scholarship. He tries to join prestigious groups and switches to smoking Parliament. After college he gets a job but is not doing well with it, and he happens to switch to Merit.

A pattern emerges: Parliament helps him mediate his blue collar past into higher society. It is a non-confrontational brand and though he has strong opinions he share those judgments privately and in acts of passive resistance. When he loses his job he is intellectually insecure and adopts Merit to boost his sense of intelligence. Perhaps he switches to **Basic** as a symbol of defiance of the middle class – a sign of going back to his roots.

Or let's take a woman who is friendly and sociable and who initiates with Virginia Slims to feel more ambitious and assertive. As she progresses with her college career and moves to a more sociable environment, she switches to **Salem**. If she spends time with a lot of men and wants to be perceived as friendlier, she might move to a man's brand or a gender-neutral brand like **Carlton** or **Merit**. In each case, the migration would reflect her movement in life.

While the identity of the smoker is an amusing parlor game at one level and perhaps a diagnostic tool at another, it becomes something completely different when smokers apply it to their own habit. Then it becomes a critical tool for the smoker who wants to quit for good. This is the issue we will explore in the next chapter.

USING PERSONAL MYTHOLOGY TO QUIT – FOR GOOD

So how does this all affect the way you quit smoking? A lot, if you are willing to take yourself and your habit apart. Smoking is revocable if you can trace your way back and, in a sense, "unsmoke." After all, you weren't born smoking, so this means that a number of issues have somehow coalesced to make you smoke.

The important first step is to separate the mental from the physical. Take your time. It is not about quitting quickly. It is about quitting completely. It could take you days or it could take years. That is not really the point. It took me four years. But when the time came, I never had an issue about going back.

So, in mythic terms, if smoking has come to fulfill the Vision Quest or a commercial path to what Joseph Campbell described as "following your bliss," then quitting must encompass it. In the absence of a replacement to the eternal coming-of-age ritual, this has become the industrialized approach to finding your path, taking your test, and being aided and rewarded by its magic powers. It follows then that no one can simply quit without resolving the "Vision Quest" issue.

Actually, the key is not so much in resolving the issue because it may not be the purpose of your life to do that; rather, it is in understanding and managing it. We turn to smoking largely to fill a void of hope and inaction. It becomes an activity, it is wish fulfillment, and it presents a binding sacrifice to a personal deity. Once you determine the psychohistory, the deity, or just the force of life you contend with, you can develop a mental smoking antidote.

The part that frightens so many quitters is the fear of putting on weight. It is actually a relatively small price to pay for giving up such a destructive habit. In fact, in may be a bit of a smokescreen for the broader issue of addiction transfer. This is what happens when you drastically interfere with an addiction without resolving the deeper issues, and so the problem simply finds another, potentially more dangerous outlet. It seems to show up most dramatically after a food addict gets a gastric bypass. Since that person is physically constricted from eating, the unresolved eating urge seeks another outlet, typically binge drinking or sexual or drug addiction. So some type of introspection is required in order to deal with the consequences of quitting and avoiding recidivism.

The difficulty with food is that the addiction may have deep roots simply because we eat from the moment of creation. At least with smoking we have a later start date. Even though smoking is traceable to the womb by way of prenatal thumb-sucking and mommy-reassurance, it is still acquired behavior and so it is easier to deconstruct. In fact, this is the safety rope of all smokers: you don't even have to resolve your issues. You can actually fake it just by going back to the moment before you became a smoker, resume that state of mind and, in a sense "unsmoke."

This is a useful trick I learned from exploring the numerous quit-smoking techniques from Jacquelyn Rogers' "You can Quit" of the nineteen seventies, the Schick Method using negative reinforcement, the nicotine replacement techniques, and the spiritual approached advocated by Deepak Chopra. It is clear from all of these approaches that any number of profound elements are at work in quitting. And yet, a simple moment of enlightenment can overcome everything, at least psychologically. This means that once you have fought that battle you are free to take on the physical addiction.

So how do you get there?

The most fascinating recent research comes from the intersection of heavy smokers, brain injury, and MRIs. If a certain part of a smoker's brain is injured that person will quit almost immediately and the addiction ceases to be an issue. According to the report in Science in January, 2007 *Jan 25, 2007 Vol. 315. no. 5811, pp. 531 – 534,* entitled "Damage to the Insula Disrupts Addiction to Cigarette Smoking" by Nasir Naqvi, David Rudrauf, Hanna Damasio, Antoine Bechara, heavy smokers who damage their insulas, a part of the brain that seems to deal with mind-body relationships, will simply stop smoking. Since no smoker would seek out a stroke or some other brain injury, such as a lesion, perhaps the weight of this book may serve the purpose of freezing the brain's myth-fulfilling bond with cigarettes.

The point of this research is that smoking has a lot more to do with the mind and soul than it does with the physical side of nicotine addiction. Arguably, the addiction is simply a way to serve the needs of the smoking mind. What we will try to do is get to the bottom of the smoking mind and try to understand why it assigns such compelling value to cigarettes. Then we will look at ways to disrupt it.

Perhaps the solution to this mystery lies in smoking's version of spontaneous remission, where people just get up one day and decide to quit. These are unquestionably lucky people because their story is the holy grail of all smokers who believe that one day they will just get up and quit. Usually, however, one finds there is more to the story: these smokers were either not really psychologically dependent or they were psychologically ready at that time, that is, whatever neuroses drove them to smoking in the first place are gone and they just no longer see the need for the habit. Unfortunately, these people are the exception, not the norm. Most smokers struggle on and off for years and then wind up with a lower tar version of what they truly bonded with.

The point is that the physical addiction, while extreme, is not all that difficult to overcome. Smokers, having built a tolerance and a residue of nicotine in their body, need to replace the missing nicotine in their bodies somewhere around one to three times an hour. Yet, as Rogers discovered in her research, it only takes three days for nicotine to leave a person's body. Some accounts vary;, for example, the student advisory from the University of Iowa in 2005 notes (http://uistudenthealth.com), that the by-products from nicotine can stay in a person's body for up to a month or more. But for the most part you could take advantage of a bad case of flu to get that nicotine out your body and theoretically you would be clean. In fact, quitting cold turkey my even feel like the flu, so you'd never know the difference.

However, almost immediately the pangs, the cravings, the insane urges will come back. In a week, that will hit you with a whammy. And in a month it only takes a whiff of someone else's smoke to find yourself reaching for a cigarette. After six months, it seems like meeting a desperately missed old friend. After a year, it is like reuniting with your old flame.

Scientists have learned that nicotine works on the brain through receptors found in various parts of the brain and even in the stomach. As a report in the Society for Neuroscience in October of 1998 Journal (sfn.org) states, "Nicotine activates a multitude of brain mechanisms by attaching to specific proteins, known as receptors, which are found on the surface of nerve cells. This interaction leads to the transmission of a chemical message. Nicotine receptors flourish in many areas of the central nervous system and diverse structural variations exist between different nicotine receptor types. Nicotine can exert dramatically different actions depending on the location and type of receptor it sticks to." These locations can even include the stomach. The net result of a satisfied receptor is the release of the happy dopamine chemicals.

While most stop-smoking advisors will tell you that the nicotine leaves the body within three days or so, there is a lot more uncertainty about the fate of those hungry nicotine receptors. It appears that they take a lot longer to fade. It is these receptors that play havoc with the quitting smoker.

The same neuroscience journal report notes that smoking may also work as medication: "Some [neuroscientists] say that a better understanding of nicotine's effects may explain why those who find it hardest to stop smoking often have other ailments such as depression or schizophrenia. These patients may be rebalancing their chemical system by treating themselves with nicotine."

For committed but otherwise normal smokers, what remains, aside from the chemical attachment, is the fact that their personal psychic order has become unhinged and no amount of medication, will power and pep talking can overcome that.

Interestingly, there are a number of techniques that use the smokers' equivalent of the Alcoholics Anonymous' approach to quit by invoking God or a higher spirit.

Deepak Chopra offers the crutch of meditation and the technique of associating the rewards of life's great things to buttress your will power when you face the cravings. At the same time, smoking is associated with a negative issue of self-image and doubt. Meditation itself can be used as a replacement for the smoking urge, but it ignores the issues of negativity: people have bad feelings and often use smoking as a way to suppress or control them. Then there is the issue of the great mythic quest, which dates back to the smoker's teenage days.

Behavior modification techniques, such as the once pioneering Schick method, is roughly similar to meditation except it uses positive and negative stimuli in place of spiritual power. But none of these really work over the long term unless you resolve issues at the source.

Rogers' smokEnders method is still a standard approach based on a 12-step method which employed a number of steps over several days or week. First, there is a preparatory step. You debrand, that is, you smoke a brand you normally detest, in order to cut down on the identification and the pleasure aspect; then you cut down on the numbers of cigarettes so there is less and less of the nicotine beast inside to feed.

At some point, when the chasm is at its narrowest, that is, when there's just a low enough amount of replacement nicotine required that you easily let go, you make that jump to nicotine freedom. But Rogers and most other methods are still prone to smokers' recidivism because the Vision Quest issue remains unresolved. Smokers get over the physical aspect but are invariably tripped up by the psychological association because they have no idea just how deep it really is.

Dealing with this issue has been complicated in the past by two issues. One issue is the simple lack of knowledge of the smoking process. The other issue is the tendency among smokers to trivialize the practice: they see it as little more than a habit that somehow gets you hooked, but is so revocable as not to be taken that seriously. The reality is much tougher because the call of youth is not merely deep, it is chthonic – it opens them up to the power of the earth. They take in these powers, its pleasures, its knowledge, and its destructive forces in blasts. They make their adjustments and build their souls and their characters and then their lives around the redux of the encounter.

As they inhale, smokers stay in touch with the cigarette's chthonic powers. Then, one day, as they respond to the sensible calls to quit, they seek a medical solution. They reach out for something rational that says, "You can give up if you just follow these steps or take these drugs." Even Zyban, which has shown great promise for treating smoking as a subset of depression and thereby providing depression replacement, will fail at this level.

So the smoker who understands that smoking is part of something that fused with his or her identity at the emergence of adulthood, is going to have to dig a lot deeper and work that much harder to beat the practice.

While one hopes that smokers begin this process as quickly as they can, it is also important to understand that it is not necessarily the fastest way to quit, because they have to work through the deeper issues. However, it is the likeliest to work in the long run. In this author's case, I have been smoke-free since 1984 and I can even light up the rare cigar without it having any residual effect on me.

When I quit back in 1984, I had given myself four years to quit. I was alone, and expected to stay that way for a long time as I worked through the research and the rejection that normally accompanies an endeavor like this book. As a young man, I didn't see my health in imminent danger and I wanted to make sure this worked for good, both the quitting and the completion of the research.

What I realized was that I hated cigarettes but I hadn't fallen out of love with tobacco. This is a very common experience because the tobacco is this great companion. It is your friend. Like Toto or the magical dog in legend - the one you see in most Disney tales - it is your friend but also your magic amulet and source of survival.

As Joseph Campbell, showed with the hero myth in "Hero With 1,000 Faces," it is an international phenomenon that exists in one form or another in every culture. It could be Moses being called by God and made to lead his people to a Promised Land where the ogre is the Pharaoh and the helper is his communication with the Almighty. It could be Jason and Argonauts, the Arthurian Legend, or the fairy tails of Grimm. The Winnebago Indians have their myths and so do any number of tribes in Africa and Asia. The common element is a calling: a special challenge, the ground rising up to meet the hero somehow delivering just the challenges he or she is uniquely suited to face.

What makes this all work is a magic enabler – often an animal, sometimes an amulet, a magic charm, or special incantation. This magic enabler has been mirrored in one way or another in smoking: tobacco takes that role and becomes your magic companion and it has to be reckoned with.

All smokers have a memory of their initial smoking experience. Often it is just about joining a group. The real question is what association did they make with the group when they undertook the private relationship necessary to learn to like smoking. This is truly the key to quitting, but you have to know both sides of the equation: what the brand stands for and what forms of empowerment it gave you, the smoker.

We know that early trauma significantly affects the way we grow up in life. Molested children often, but not always, grow up to be molesters or violent people. Typical therapy requires the uncovering of the original trauma and deactivating the chain of consequences, and substituting where possible a new program of responses. Even money management has been shown to reflect early trauma. Suze Orman, the financial advisor, has built a large following by identifying that peoples' earliest experiences with money not only affects the way they deal with money in later life but even their sense of self-esteem.

The critical point is that original associations compound over time and generate secondary associations. To complicate matters, the whole process is submerged in the unconscious and people lose knowledge – and with that, control - over the process.

So what are the equivalent cigarette memories and how are they a factor in quitting?

Since the habit of smoking is often clouded by memories of starting as part of a group, people tend to overlook the personal motivation. But there is always a personal motivation and the key to finding it is to identify the originating brand and its specific role in establishing your adult identity. It is extremely difficult, if not impossible, for a committed smoker to quit without coming to terms with this in one way or another. Once the source is identified it is possible to understand the nature of the Vision Quest and then the psychic strategy of quitting can begin.

The physical act of smoking is relatively straight-forward and can be eradicated through the method of your choosing: cold turkey, a debranding and winding down of the habit before jumping the chasm, a form of positive and negative stimuli, a spiritual withdrawal, or a nicotine replacement.

Resolving the "inner" issue is a different story. Whether or not you accept the idea that smokers are responding to a coming-**out** or challenge by submitting themselves to a kind of mythic force, we do know there is a start date and some kind of impetus, not just to start smoking, but to go to the effort of becoming a smoker, which is unpleasant and can take about three weeks.

Resolving that issue begins with that step back in time to the initiation period; specifically, to the private times the smoker had to spend "learning" or acclimating him or herself to the initially unpleasant practice of smoking. The typical personal issues that trigger smoking among teenagers include significant lack of self-esteem, depression, fear of sexual inadequacy, gender uncertainty, fear of ugliness, or even self-mutilation as a response to early trauma. Indeed, there are as many reasons as there are variations in the human condition. Whatever the teen trigger, it has to be confronted by the adult smoker who may or may not have moved on from the issues they struggled with as a teen. Nevertheless, years of psychological associations, and even benefits, have been established on that base. It can't simply be abandoned. In simple terms, it then has to be undone either through being transferred to something else or, if a smoker is so lucky that the original issues have been resolved, then simply acknowledged and put at rest. In either case, it requires a specific counter ritual for most people.

The great secret to quitting smoking, at least quitting for good, lies right here. If you pick a replacement ritual that improves you, this not only protects you from recidivism but it takes you to a higher level as a human being. This may well be the secret to quitting all kinds of addictive behaviors but it certainly applies with smoking and explains why heavy smokers who quit often describe it as the greatest achievement in their lives. Or at least, the one of which they are proudest.

One way to develop a counter ritual is to think of the techniques used successfully in hypnotherapy. Typically, in hypnotherapy, key ideas and phrases are taken from the subject during analysis and crafted into messages that are delivered to the subject under hypnosis. This can be a powerful tool that has a special relevance to smoking, which, as we indicated, creates a sense of well-being in smokers that roughly equates to a trance. Since smoking is a replacement for an activity or state of mind that the smoker as a teen was once unable to attain. The key is to fashion a counter ritual out of that path the teenage smoker was unable to take so that the psychological addiction can be overcome.

In my case, at the physical level, I focused on how I could have gone for a karate black belt but didn't and then embarked on journey to one. Then I took the time-honored approach of tobacco replacement - moving from cigarettes, first to cigars, and then to tobacco pouches, which had the effect of displacing cigarette nicotine with less convenient forms of tobacco that are much easier to deal with and resist. It was like going from crack to less addictive forms until ultimately quitting - for good.

Fortunately, with this approach, it is relatively easy to stay away from cigarettes once you substitute for them, since they contain so many additives. Once you move from cigarettes and the nicotine is absorbed from alternate means, it often is hard to return to cigarettes per se because the additives become identifiable and distasteful. At that point, the movement to non-cigarette nicotine delivery products is easy and in turn it tends to be easier to quit non-cigarette addiction because the alternate products don't offer all the features of cigarette that give it its psychological well-being; they are less convenient, less nicotine is absorbed, and less of the ritual accompanies the practice. The key is that the smoker has to move in a deliberate passage from cigarette smoking to isolating the practice of nicotine absorption. On its own, nicotine addiction can be overcome in about three days.

As the process of isolating nicotine absorption from smoking continues, this is the special period where smokers can separate out the spiritual side of their practice and come to terms with it. Naturally, it is important in physical habit terms to use the quitting techniques that provide alternatives like chewing gum or munching on carrots. It also helps to employ strategies like drinking water or diet soda.

But the key we are after, is to understand the quest and the assistance that tobacco provides.

By retracing your footsteps you are being asked what psychological value smoking provided you. At this point, your knowledge of the brands should give you that clue. The crux of the exercise is to determine the specific issue – outside of joining a group for which the brand offered a benefit. Did you smoke **Marlboro** because you wanted to join the group of tough guys and **Marlboro** eased your path by putting you in touch with the warrior inside? Did Camel make you overcome your sexual problems or was smoking a mask for those problems? Did Virginia Slims buttress your sense of defiance as you entered college and began your path to law school? Did **Winston** give you courage to face a team of opponents? Did **Salem** make you feel more powerful than you were? Did your brand make you feel prettier, more special?

After defining the specific power, you have to devise a strategy to deal with the spirit power of the brand working back to the initiation brand. At the symbolic level, it is important to devise the right ceremony that works for you. It could be as simple as a mock wake or a trip to a special place remembered from your youth. This also requires a replacement strategy like learning a new skill or sport. In my case I trained for a black belt in Tae Kwon Do. But I could have chosen anything: tennis, competitive tennis, track, cycling, or skiing. The important thing is that this replacement strategy should have a special significance – preferably a skill that for some reason was suppressed at youth.

The reason this is important is because these mythic exchanges typically demand a quid pro quo. In primitive storytelling the payment for release is usually dire and drenched with violence or some unspeakable practice. For example, in the Bible, Joseph worked for seven years in return for marrying the wrong daughter; in order to marry the right one, he had to work seven more years. In the M'swati myth of West Africa, in return for helping a starving woman, the lightening god demands to marry her first born if she turns out to be a girl. The first born turns out to be a girl and when the lightning god comes to demands his prize, the woman has long forgotten this oath. Naturally, she resists and tragedy ensues. At the personal level, the psyche similarly demands a heavy payment for giving up its part of the deal. Ignoring or resisting this demand usually sparks a return to smoking; you have no defense other than to go back to smoking.

Let's take the example of a young white musician who adopts Kool to feel comfortable among fellow black musicians. In this case a payback strategy and replacement technique might entail doing a charity effort for inner city kids or a special act to understand the struggles of African Americans.

We know why cultures throughout the world have developed mythology – it is a precursor to religion to help them explain their lives. The revelation is that myth and religion have so many common elements. And although they offer roughly similar explanations about our existence on earth and the world of divinity, there are key differences between modern religion and ancient tribalism. Most native cultures also provide a way to reach the supernatural world, typically involving a trance dance, imbibing of beer or spirits or a psychoactive substance. we in the West may use prayer in an attempt to do the same thing but prayer rarely involves the altering of consciousness. For that we rely on what we consider the vices, including liquor, drugs, and, to some extent, tobacco. Only hypnotherapy seems to visit this area without being considered a vice. However, when we do enter the world of vices we are taking a step back in time where the rules are much closer to the ones of the ancient world and where we must act accordingly.

The lure of cigarettes is that they do all of that in a modern way, and when we throw them aside we need to deconstruct the process, go back to the source, and find a substitute or reparative myth and pay whatever symbolic dues are owed for changing course.

Deepak Chopra, who himself had been a smoker, views all addictions as a kind of misdirected quest for spirituality. As a consequence, he recommends a spiritual path of redemption with includes regular meditations. By the same token, it is entirely possible to use the Alcoholics Anonymous' approach and bring the Almighty to bear on the problem. Chopra used the associative process, that is, using positive associations such as imagining the good moments in his life, to help him deal with the smoking pangs. What makes his method more powerful is that it is backed with meditation.

Most people, however, will still have to confront the essential issue of what the tobacco meant to their Vision Quest. Without confronting this issue, the seduction of cigarettes is simply too strong. Even Mark Twain faced this, saying that "Quitting smoking is easy, I've done it hundreds of times." Recidivism has always been the great bogeyman of smoking cessation. Even today, the best programs have a 50% failure rate and the average program remains in the 70-80% recidivism range. Understanding the Vision Quest and resolving the psychic bond are the missing pieces of the puzzle.

Summary of the Personal Mythology Approach

Not everyone can look at their smoking history from the inside. Introspection is a tough challenge for the average person, even if it is presented as a kind of "personal backtracking." So there is another – an external way - to solve the puzzle of the initiation brand, and that is to look at it from the outside: what does it mean to the smoker and what was the "Vision Quest" it offered that person or what practice did it "enable" him to follow? For example, if as a teen this smoker loved car racing and smoked **Winston** to be "one of the boys," then he has a great start.

There are two approaches to solving this problem:

Approach One: Determine the relationship of the smoker to the brand – to understand what the brand "does" for him or her.

You begin with this question: Does the smoker match the brand?

If the answer is yes, then the issue is that the image fuels that smoker and he or she needs to find a steady alternative. However, it is also important to ask whether the smoker matched the brand when he or she started. In other words, we are asking what was this particular smoker's relationship back then and did he grow into the brand? The personal growth is either strong enough to go on without the brand or that smoker is going to need a replacement that roughly matches the psychic support of the brand. Typically, the replacement is a sport or an activity that fills that role. The more active the replacement, the better the chance of quitting.

If the answer is no, and the image and the smoker are out of synch, then the issue is finding out what the smoker is compensating for and determining what the brand really brings to the table. Sometimes determining the value of the brand is highly personal and would be interpreted in the same way a dream symbol is done – by using an association test. The smoker lists his or her associations to the brand image and the replacement therapy is based on finding the resonant image and replacing it. Once again, the issues typically relate to sex, status, self-esteem, or rejuvenation.

Approach Two: Relive the days of youth when the smoker began smoking. What were the conditions, how did his or her brand history evolve? Can this smoker remember why he selected that brand and what he hoped to achieve? If the answer is not obvious, then we have to take Approach One and apply it to the person they were when they began smoking. If that smoker matched the brand, an active replacement is relatively straightforward. If there was no match to the brand, then the challenge is more significant but by no means insurmountable. In essence, that smoker has to reinvent his or her life history from the point of view of an imaginary life. For instance, if they hoped to be tougher, more adventurous, or more assertive, he has to pick an activity that addresses this need and allows them to re-imagine and continue their life without smoke. I know of people who dreamt of being mountain climbers who used the climbing wall as a safe way to satisfy the fantasy and give them a proactive means of quitting.

Using the Cigarette Seduction Brand Knowledge to Quit
This approach to quitting entails three parts: **Will**, **Ritual** and **Technique**.

Step 1. You have to want to quit. Will power is important but it only goes so far. The *desire* to quit along with a substantive technique is the way to quit. Brand knowledge helps you customize the technique for your specific psychic needs.

Step 2. You make an honest assessment of the psychic power of the brand and develop a replacement strategy**,** e.g., sports or other physical activity with deep meaning, along with a ritual for marking the stages of that effort. The rituals need not be hard – just accessible. For example, if, after all these years, you decide to play tennis because once you dreamed of playing in the U,S. Open, then the ritual may just be about qualifying to play at a certain level. Or perhaps you once dreamed about getting certified for scuba diving, learning the butterfly stroke, making a promise to play at every major golf course in the northeast, or even something like achieving a higher level of skiing at every major resort in Colorado.

Breathing and the Ritual. The ritual only has to be significant from the perspective of resolving the Vision Quest issue and the brand issue should have provided the key to understanding that issue. In order to be most effective, the ritual should have a physical aspect or at least some feature relating to breathing. Since breath power is a key part of smoking, there is no question that it is helpful to learn deep breathing techniques. The simplest approach to diaphragm breathing that is often used in the martial arts is to contract the sphincter muscles and breathe deeply. This technique also helps a person to deal with stress.

Milestones. It is also important to adopt ritual milestones that roughly match the stages of quitting:
• Three days when the nicotine leaves the body
• One week when the urge returns with a vengeance
• One month when you gravitate to picking it up the habit again without thinking
• Six months when you feel like testing yourself and
• One year later when you are tempted to do it "for old time's sake,"

Step 3. Adopt a cessation strategy. With all the other pieces in place you can pick your approach. The classic smokEnders technique (e.g. debranding, cutting down, and quitting) the aided version (a patch, a pill like Zyban, or tobacco substitute gum), my lazy man version with cigars and chewing tobacco, hypnosis (especially effective if it incorporates the Vision Quest information), or just plain cold turkey quitting. In fact, most people adopt some combination of the above; often, they use additional aids, including drinking a lot of water, chewing carrots and celery, or drinking coffee.

Optional Step 4. Develop a closing ceremony. Many authorities suggest buying yourself a special gift or perhaps taking a special trip **or e**ven going back to school. As long as this method ties in with the Vision Quest issue, it is a very good idea to reward yourself with something special.

More About the Mythology of Quitting

The hardest thing about quitting is making the committed decision to stop. There is so much to give up: the companionship, the habit, the rituals, and that intangible thing - the powerful, indescribable element which is the psychic power you derive from smoking.

To really quit, you need a strategy.

Most quitting techniques work on the idea of narrowing the gap between your dependence and the world of abstinence. These techniques focus on making the chasm seem like a simple step. But a chasm, no matter how narrow, is still a chasm and it is always scary.

It helps if you believe you can jump. Quitting is an almost guaranteed success if you take on the psychology of a successful quitter even before you've taken the leap. But that only works if you have a complete belief system that helps you understand the "afterlife" of your world without smoking.

The best way to do this it by understanding the psychic support you're getting from your brand, that is the brand knowledge can help understand the personal mythic story it supports. Then you need a conversion strategy: a way to transfer the psychic life support system to other grounds, a way of living in abstinence without feeling like it is abstinence. In other words, the idea of self-sufficiency without any thought of cigarettes.

A life without smoking.

If the psyche is prepared, the physical drudgery of quitting is reduced to a pleasant if occasionally challenging exercise. The fact is, if the psyche is prepared, life is made easier for the person quitting.

It happens enough as a natural occurrence that most struggling quitters feel they ought to experience it as a birthright. What most smokers seem to look for is an opening or a sign that they are ready to quit. If they are not stuck by a sudden change in psyche then they feel they're just not ready to quit.

But you can learn how to master the smoking psyche.

So another way of looking at this technique is that it helps you to discover the "magic moment." You can take your time if you have to. But having a technique gives you faith. Then you can use the technique with any quit-smoking program.

Expressed in a slightly different way, these are three basic steps.

1. Identify the Initiation Bond.

What made you initially connect with smoking and a particular brand? This connection will typically reflect a time of teenage angst. This connection is the critical element that ties you to smoking and makes quitting easier once you understand it. Knowing what the brand of your youth meant to you can help you get to the bottom of your smoking attachment.

2. Develop a Psychic Replacement Strategy

You don't have to solve all your emotional problems to quit. You only have to develop a way of facing them without smoking. Typically, an activity that you wanted to do as a teen but were not able to - especially one that smoking seemed to prohibit, like sports or some kind of excercise - works well.

3. Take On a Ritual

When you quit smoking, a kind of companion dies. You need a ritual that keeps it that way and gives you a sense of afterlife in your post-smoking world. If you combine an activity, for example, competitive tennis or karate, with a ritual, such as regular activity or a mantra, this method will work so much better.

4. Optional: A Closing Reward Ritual

When you feel that you have achieved smoke cessation get yourself a very special gift that memorializes the process as well as celebrates the victory. The ideal gift could well be a hiking tour or a workout center, but, in any case, the general principle is any activity or gift that requires a good breathing capability.

You could almost say that the right ritual is everything. No question, finding a practice you desire that could only be achieved after quitting provides a huge incentive to quit. This method definitely works with overweight people who have been offered a chance to appear on TV in a swim suit; the public is amazed to find how much they are willing to diet and exercise. Granted that is temporary but it is a start. The best method involves a practice that has a deep, special meaning for you.

Most smokers have a ritual connection to their brand that traces back to their very first choice. The clue is not so much the first cigarette as it is the first cigarette they bonded with – after all, the first cigarette probably made you puke. Typically, there is a coded association between a smoker's teenage angst and the brand they chose at that time. The total experience is a kind of ritual that can be taken apart and resolved.

When they are digging up the past, smokers may find they have outgrown many of the issues associated with the brand. Simple problems such as "I am not tough enough.... not pretty enough...sophisticated enough..." may have ceased being a issue as they have grown up, but they forgot that the issue still underlies their smoking. If that is the case, then once you get to the bottom of that issue, the added overlay of habit and daily ritual can be thrown off like a crust.

Unfortunately, most cases are not that simple, so somehow the needs persist or the issues have morphed. If the insecurities exist, then understanding the origin tells you where you are today in contrast to where you where then. The challenge is to devise an alternative ritual.

Using Nervous Energy

Quitting usually throws off nervous energy, which can easily be counter-productive. So, the trick is to find foods and activities that not only replace but also take advantage of the extra energy thrown off by quitting. If you do this, you will fare well. But if the activity takes on a special meaning as part of a ritual then you will do even better.

One of the challenges is that when you quit smoking you are giving up a kind of friend. You can get depressed. You may feel like something has died because something is missing, something has been taken from you. You will also find yourself gaining back the time you once wasted on standing around smoking. You don't want to squander that; this extra healthy energy should be used as a bonus.

Resolving the Vision Quest

On a deeper level, however, at the mythic form of ritual, when you began smoking, you were making a deal with a higher being so that if you endured some punishment – as a kind of challenge – you would gain psychic power. This is usually a lifelong arrangement. You don't abandon the arrangement without incurring the wrath of the "higher beings." So you either have to make a deal or find another power to help you oppose the first higher being. In other words, the new activity has to be a working response to this issue and it also has to be captured in ritual. That returns power to the quitter and fortifies him or her during moments of doubt.

Take the example of a teenager who feared that he would be unloved by women and finds that smoking gives him just enough of an edge to win over women,- or, at least, so he believes. If he also finds that he gets this edge best with the Camel brand, then our challenge is not just about pointing that out. He also has to find an activity and some type of ritual that makes him feel as much of an attraction as he did with Camel. That could mean playing tennis and then dressing especially well, while evolving a new kind of attitude and even a new way of thinking about himself.

A riskier approach would be involved if the smoker found that smoking Carlton as a teenager was associated with his sense of being oppressed, or he smoked **Newport** because he didn't think he was affluent enough. Then the replacement activity would probably involve something ego-boosting or challenging; something like skydiving, downhill cycling, competitive swimming, or even taking on a new career or extra-curricula activity such as helping the poor. Again, the activity will probably work if it is also somehow ritualized.

The cessation ritual is typically a repetitive act that is often accompanied and certainly aided by a phrase or message that gives reassurance to the quitter – something like a mantra. The deeper the ritual's attachment with the sense of self, the more profound the effect.

When a person accepts a ritual, it is much less likely for him or her to slip back if the ritual is properly structured and puts the issue of psychological identity into play. Naturally, the more physical the activity the better, because turning back to smoking will immediately undermine the new activity and force the ex-smoker to confront him or herself. If the smoker's mental commitment is good, he's get over his past actions easily, bonding with the new activity. Any activity, from knitting to walking the dog is good, but the activity is always better if it relates to breathing.

For example, a smoker might feel that his impulse as a teen was to cover up his deficiencies in competitive sports, so he begins smoking **Winston**. Twenty years later he could take up tennis as a regular activity and as a typically sociable **Winston**ite, spend more time in the clubhouse along with playing tennis. He has an advantage now because being older means that there are fewer **Players** around and people are therefore more welcoming and less competitive, so it is easier to establish self-esteem The key is to accept the tennis experience as part of the replacement ritual and to try to bond with it. Hanging around in the clubhouse is fine, as long as it doesn't lead to the temptation to smoke.

So long as the specific quitting technique works with your personality it is doesn't matter which one you choose. One key issue, however, is that you have a plan to deal with the crisis points in quitting that typically occur around the following times:

• The third day, when the nicotine leaves your system;

• The first week, when you *must* have a cigarette (remember it takes time for the nicotine receptors to fade);

• The first month, when you think you can have just one for old time's sake; and

• About six months, when you feel your personality hasn't really adapted to the loss of smoking.

Any form of tapering off or negative or positive reinforcement to break the habit can work. However, only when the psychic attachment is resolved does it really work - it is then easier to quit completely. And when you are off smoking because you are being psychically nourished elsewhere, there is just no reason to go back. There is nothing pulling you, nothing to tempt you. There is no cigarette seduction.

You are free.

Welcome to the New World Without Smoke

When we can't solve a problem our instinct is to tax it. So when the great moral showdown came between society and the tobacco barons in 1997, it turned out be an attorney general's day at the races followed by a windfall for politicians. The settlement's $25 billion annual price tag was way beyond the imaginations of anybody in the public health field. So was the rapidity of the solution – just two years.

At the end of the day, the solution was based on taxing the smoker while handing out a pittance to the health officials charged with keeping teens off tobacco. The overwhelming bulk of the monies have gone to fill road projects and budget gaps.

There are many possible criticisms of the deal and the roles of the various participants. The tobacco companies know their customers are addicted and will pay almost anything to keep on smoking. So the tobacco executives were glad to pay (with their customers - the smokers' - money) to stave off any threat of criminal action pertaining to things like perjury – such as lying before Congress about whether nicotine was addictive.

The health groups were generally against any kind of settlement that didn't result in the indictments of tobacco executives. The only time the health groups appeared satisfied was when the attorneys general dropped immunity from class action from the settlement, thus allowing various parties to keep badgering the tobacco companies with class action suits.

The health groups had little real leverage in the settlement and their hunger for punishment kept them far from the innards of the tobacco companies – great profitable institutions with hundreds of thousands of employees seeking an honorable place in the society of citizens.

While the tiny amount the health groups have received from the settlement – no more than 5%, and in many states, nothing at all – it is still more money than they have gotten from the tobacco issue in the past. The real problem for the health groups is that they have no strategy of engagement with the tobacco companies other than to vilify both them and the practice of smoking.

While the tobacco companies are certainly deserving of opprobrium, the real issue is what strategies they have to deal with the smoking phenomenon if, as we are discovering, it is more than just a function of tobacco companies cramming it down the throats of teens. There is an underlying phenomenon driving teens into their arms. Not all teens and not all the time - but there are enough teens coming on a regular basis who are also impervious to the negative appeals or to the dramatic increases in price. Their appetite is inexorable and they just keep coming.

We see this as the peculiar expression of the primitive coming of age ritual often spurred on by depression or some other personal issue ranging from social insecurity to lack of self-esteem. The question is what can we do to transform this terrible issue?

While there is every reason to go on bashing the tobacco business, the real answer lies in dealing with the issue in its true perspective. Smoking is a lot more revocable now that we have some devices and medical approaches to make quitting so much easier than it was years ago. So, as bad as smoking may be, it is not quite the death sentence it was back in the olden days when most people just couldn't quit.

We know that if smoking satisfies certain needs then, all the negative smoking billboards in the world will make little difference over the long run without an alternative, without a real working response to those needs. Teens will always turn to something destructive. It may be smoking, or it may be worse, including enlisting in the military. Wars, after all, cannot be fought without 18-year olds.

While **Cigarette Seduction** is primarily focused on relatively normal teens who are attracted to smoking because it promises a kind of initiation, there is plenty of evidence that survival of smoking as practice is being fueled by a population that sees it as a kind of psychic medicine. Studies such as reported in a paper in the American Journal of Psychiatry in the September, 2003, *American Journal of Psychiatry 160:1663-1669*] shows that smokers today are now more than three times likely to be depressed than non-smokers. Some studies claim that as much as half of smokers are depressed or have some type of mental pathology. Teens may simply be in one of "those phases" and find themselves ineluctably drawn toward smoking. The morally-laden "Just say no" or "Oh my god, look at your lungs thirty years from now" stuff just isn't going to cut it if teens are driven by psychic pain.

We're really talking about society's most popular medication against the pain of living. Society once supported this product as a standard practice, even putting it in our soldier's "K" rations. By the mid-twentieth century over half of Americans smoked. Now the number of smokers is dropping but society hasn't come up with a substitute. To many kids, smoking just seems like a prescription for righteous rebellion!

Our main concern is less about "just say no" and more about ensuring that teens are less likely to be stuck with smoking for life, not just as tobacco users but as addicts. If smoking is truly revocable, or something that could be dabbled with and then easily dropped, much of the health danger will be diminished. Ultimately, the health workers' mission is about saving peoples' lives and not making moral decisions. For that reason, the concern should be about what we can do to help teens get through the Vision Quest period without locking them into lifetime of asphyxiation.

In its simplest form, we need to have a comprehensive approach to give teens deep strategies for dealing with their passage into life. Simply saying no is just not good enough. It isn't even close.

When we consider the key instigators for smoking, including joining a new group, overcoming depression, managing sexual identity, increasing self-esteem, managing a weight issue or perceived ugliness, we need a working strategy to help teen smokers deal with instigators at each level and for each problem. Some of these issues are truly grave and need to be dealt with accordingly, not sloughed off with a "just say no" campaign. Others are more behavioral, for example, the overweight person looking for a way to feel she can control their weight while making her condition seem more acceptable to others. So the way to treat these issues may be oral substitutes or real weight management products other than smoking. If depression is a factor, it should be treated medically. There is even an argument that the gum industry ought to develop a "serious" gum, something that would match the oral satisfaction and image projection a pack of cigarettes gives.

Some issues only society can decide: do we make it easy for medical professionals to prescribe teen smokers drugs or at least find youngsters who are in need a real substitute? Do we listen to the call of the soul and find Vision Quests that satisfy teens' need to transition in adulthood? Do we ignore these needs and offer kids simple pieties or do we just keep blaming the tobacco companies and encourage kids to vent against them? This is not an entirely bad approach but it does not solve the problem of teen motivation for smoking; it doesn't deal with what drives them to want to smoke.

Naturally, the aim of this game is to keep teens from smoking. But there really is no overall benefit to society if teens wind up doing something more harmful instead. What we really want is a solution that motivates them to quit rather than forces them into it. At the same time, their psychic needs have to be satisfied, or they will go elsewhere.

To some extent we already have this in the form of sports. But that is also a limited spectrum; not everyone can participate meaningfully in sports nor does it offer all the necessary complexity. Besides, these are appointment activities and we are looking for an everyday, whole life experience that addresses the deep issues of the soul.

Fortunately, we understand that there is money out there from the tobacco settlement and a moral obligation to dedicate some of that money to this cause, and that could make a huge difference. But we still have to face this cause – the Vision Quest – that deals with the deeper issues that smoking appears to address.

Oddly, the greatest danger for the anti-smoking movement is the newfound, if grudging, respect society is willing to give the tobacco industry. Keep in mind, the tobacco companies are now huge contributors to 50 state budgets and over time that point will not be forgotten by the states' politicians. The main fear, however, is innovation. Suppose the tobacco companies come to the conclusion that their real mission is to find the next solutions to the Vision Quest problem and market their products accordingly. Suppose they make their products safe enough to pass muster with sensitive lawmakers. Suppose they make some new version of smoking that appears acceptable to our known science only to create a long-term hazard that only future generations will discover? Maybe the tobacco companies will jump on the "nicotine is good for you" bandwagon by delivering it in a non-carcinogenic manner. For example, **Blue Whale**, a chewing tobacco that has no tobacco but plenty of nicotine just might be a step in that direction. Or the tobacco industry may get medical on us. If so, since a number of mental pathologies appear to be served by smoking, maybe they'll come up with a line of prescription smokes. The one sure thing about medication-by-smoking is that you don't have to worry about your patients forgetting to take their meds. Nicotine is one of those drugs that insures that patients take their dosage like clockwork.

In one of my slightly ironic articles I point out how few of the teenage mass-murderers smoke, but often turn to shooting after giving up their doctor-prescribed medication. If we combined smoking with medication, this would almost certainly not be an issue!

How Come School Shooters Don't Seem to Smoke?

[These tragedies suggest this chillingly cogent argument - should cigarettes be considered a form of self-medication? Or, since cigarettes are addictive and consumed like clockwork - whereas most shooters are set off because they quit their antidepressants - should not the two should be combined?]

After the horrific shootings, there is always a swarm of agents with alphabet soup windbreakers that rummage through the wreckage. Leading this group is the BATF, Bureau of Alcohol, Tobacco and Firearms, which is generally there to find casings and match them to the weapons.

It's hard to imagine how much difference this information will make since we already know who the shooter was and just how legally they got their top of the line weapon technology.

So why aren't they making good use of their time on the "A" and the "T" - looking for alcohol bottles and discarded cigarette butts? Granted, psychopaths seem to shun alcohol on their highly organized trails of retribution. But what about cigarettes?

Good and bad people - even sober judges - smoke. So how come there never seems to be a trail of smoldering butts? No unfinished **Marlboro**s to mark their High Noon moment? Never a cruel cigarillo to show their contempt for society and its second-hand smoke regulations?

This is not just the Virginia Tech killer, the mad boys of Columbine seemed to be similarly abstemious. Then there is the shooting at Pearl, Miss., Jacksboro, Tenn. - and even the Amish country schoolhouse where I just can't think of any one of them puffing on a stick, Bogey-like. John Hinckley shot Reagan with nary a puff, ditto for Chapman with John Lennon.

It seems like bad form to talk cigarettes at a time like this, although Virginia Tech's shooter Cho, did mention Hitler, and Hitler as we know, was a non-smoker. (A vegetarian too, but that is another issue).

Is this to suggest that smoking a pack or two a day might have helped? Maybe - studies like the St. Louis survey and a recent American Journal of Psychiatry paper show that smoking and depression are profoundly linked.

The Secret Service psychologist, Dr. Robert Fein, in his study of stalkers and assassins, called the "Exceptional Case Study," agrees. He adds there is another connected and recurring issue in the profiles of these diverse killers – with the possible exception of Hitler: that they were all at first suicidal. Once they had accepted their own demise, everything else in their terrible quests seemed to fit in rather nicely.

Now cigarettes, that much maligned flourish of youth, have the reputation, at least as far as former secretary of Health, Education, and Welfare Joseph A. Califano, Jr. is concerned, as being little more than a form of slow-motion suicide. Normally, you'd agree - who wants to be suicidal? But now we know what suicidal and depressed people can do once you free them of their bad habits, smoking may not be such a terrible thing after all.

Most reports, including those on the ASH.org website will tell you that 88% or so, of smokers have started by age 18. Except for these fellows, of course. (And it usually is fellows.) Obviously, smoking serves as a much needed form of initiation and these outcasts seem to have missed the boat.

Maybe we should invite them back. There's something to be said for the idea of troubled people taking their suicide in slow, twenty minute increments rather than letting go in a hail of gunfire. Second-hand smoke may be a small price to pay. Besides, these shooters tend have been prescribed antidepressants but then stop taking their meds. That never happens with smokers – once they're hooked they keep taking their smokes like clockwork.

So maybe we need to rethink the value of smoking. Of course, this would take some revisionist compromising. But dusting off the old "Reach for a Lucky Instead of a Glock" campaign is worth another look. And Lucky Strikes could be a good thing in a world of calculating psychopaths. Kool could have done just that - cooled a killer down. Camel - that could have meant nothing more than a trip to the zoo.

Realistically though, our current cigarette brands aren't quite suicidal enough. We may have to develop a more compelling, more clinically informed family of brands that communicate the idea: "Why shoot me when you could be smoking one of these bad boys?"

This is not necessarily a call for the resurrection of the tobacco companies. After all, Philip Morris recently left New York in a puff as mounting taxes and regulation seemed to pull the rug under their Park Ave. welcome. So they moved their headquarters back to Richmond, Virginia which didn't help the situation anyway. Apparently, easy guns trump easy cigarettes.

What we really need are prescription-strength cigarettes that health professionals can custom-design for troubled souls. We could call them Cig-Rx. They could have clinical names like Pufficide DX, or 2 Paxil-a-Day. Or they could go to the heart of the problem with displacement fantasy brands like Death Rays, Anti-Harmony, Bad Deeds, My Punishment and the freshly mentholated, Unhappy Days. These solutions are cheap, generate taxes and nourish our farmlands.

All of this really happening anyway, we just don't control it properly. Psychcentral.com reports that doctors Cheong, Herkov & Goodman found in the St. Louis study, that depressed smokers use their cigarettes quite successfully as a way to self-medicate. This approach appears to be growing. A September 2003 study in the American Journal of Psychiatry (160:1663-1669), shows that smokers today are now more 3 times likely to be depressed than non-smokers. This is a relatively new phenomenon: back when smoking was widely accepted, there was no significant difference in depression rates between smokers and non-smokers.

Twenty five years ago that all began to change. Fewer people were smoking, but those who did were more like likely to be depressed. Note how that coincides with the beginning of this wave of suicidal, depressed, well-armed and non-smoking killers with Chapman in 1980 and Hinckley in 1981. Could it be that the health movement got to the wrong people? If so, could they call off the dogs and let them smoke again. Could the troubled people just blow off their steam again, please. It may not be good for their lungs but it could save my life. If that didn't work at least their aura of smoke and puffing would serve as an early warning system. If you could at least smell them coming, the head start alone might be worth all the horses in **Marlboro** Country.

The point about any of these scenarios is that the health groups, for the most part, have "just said no." Yet, if the tobacco companies solve any of these problems, they get to own the future and public health takes a back seat, just as it did for most of the last century.

Smoking has to change, if for no other reason than tobacco companies have to find ways to keep their customers. White-collar smokers already face an untenable situation at work because they have to go out of the office every time they want to smoke. That could amount to as many as three trips during an hour. Aside from the disruptions, it means that the smokers are losing 10 or 15 minutes an hour of work.

Employers, too, are coming to realize that they are not getting full value from their smoking staff since they have to take off about 10-5 minutes of every hour for their smoking breaks. In a sense, smokers are getting paid a psychiatrist's 45-minute hour and this situation is likely to come to a head as the economy moves closer to a real recession. Suddenly, employers will start to think about refusing to hire smokers because of their lost productivity.

If you are not sure about the way this works, you have only to look at the smokers congregated outside their office smoking area. No matter how cold it is, the men never wear coats and oftentimes not even a jacket. The women seem to favor cardigans. Why? Because they don't want to signal to their bosses that they are leaving for a smoke. How long before employers discount smokers' work time by the number of smoke breaks they take?

At first, that may be a good thing for the anti-smoking movement. But in the long run it could be the worst thing because it will force innovation. No one quits smoking if their psychological need remains unfulfilled. So smokers will start to buy patches or other forms of ingested tobacco, not for the purpose of quitting but to keep them satisfied while they stretch out the time between smoke breaks at work. Right now, the drug companies are selling patches to help people quit. But since these patches can't resolve the psychological issues, and here we really means the ones that cross into the kind of spiritual/psychic space discussed in most of this book, then the patches will start to be sold as a kind of cigarette helper, a device that salves the monkey on your back until the coast is truly clear.

So, who would be the best marketers of that product?

You guessed it. But that would put the tobacco companies into a line of business that looks a lot like a branch of the health industry. Since the tobacco companies still have a huge flow of income this then opens the door for the companies to use that money to get into the business of smokers life-coping skills. It would behoove them to develop a slew of nicotine patch, gum, spray, and even nicotine water companies of their own, thereby essentially turning smoke cessation into more of a smoke management business.

The tobacco companies may suddenly find that the public has developed a new interest in the so-called safe cigarettes and nicotine delivery devices that the companies have they put years of research into and embrace them in the same way they once embraced filter tips over plain tips or low tar over regular cigarettes. Filters were around for a long time before the cancer scare made them desirable.

As the public understanding of the psychodynamics of smoking increases, so might its sympathy for the practice and its real story. The laws may change to accommodate the practices based around a low smoke emission product or a nicotine delivery system. Indeed, genetic engineering may yield a nicotine- like product that delivers the special qualities smokers seek, particularly the slight lift and the sense of appeasing the discomfort of a powerful internal ache with a psychic friend.

If the products no longer issue second-hand smoke, then tobacco or its natural successor is likely to be welcomed back in the workplace. If it is perceived as less carcinogenic, millions will revisit the habit. Most of all, the moral authority and the moment of public suasion and visibility of the health movement will pass. Their voice of conscience and good health will drift into irrelevancy.

A somehow cleansed tobacco industry that is perceived as no worse and perhaps even more welcome than say, the beer industry, is a powerful beast indeed. Few businesses generate the industry's cash flow or the sheer regularity of its revenues. In five years they could grow not only in power but this time they will have cheering group in the form of state and federal governments dependent on cigarette taxes. In the end, we may witness a kind of turning the clock back to the World War II years when tobacco was considered to be a strategic product for the war effort.

The extraordinary advantage the tobacco companies have is the allegiance of their customers, who are much too attached to their products to do anything but stay on. That gives tobacco companies a high probability of succeeding with innovations and even reinventing themselves as a new kind of life-coping management industry. After all, weren't financial planners once just door-to-door life insurance salesmen?

Health groups need to take a leadership role in the development of life management skills for people who may be at risk of becoming or who may already become smokers. At the simplest level this could be a program to certify and reward teens who don't smoke. After all, what teen wants to be a goody-two-shoes for nothing? More importantly, health groups have to get over the image of moral superiority based on the idea that what they advocate is "good for you" so that not smoking should be its own reward. That attitude gives the tobacco companies a huge advantage as they provide identity, pleasure, the Vision Quest, and catalogs of free merchandise for dedicated smokers, and sponsor events like concerts and parties that teens crave. The health movement, on the other hand, even with an attitude, is like your vegetables, just good for you with no immediately tangible rewards.

The health movement might improve its impact if they also gave away premiums *for not smoking.* Giving goodies is a small thing, but it is a start, especially if the "goodies" inherently promote healthy activities and can be sponsored by sports equipment, sports drink, or vitamin companies.

The most powerful development, and the one necessary to keep the movement relevant over the long run, is a giant task that cannot be taken lightly: the willingness to enter the business of developing and managing the Vision Quest of teens. This would have to start as early as age 10 or 11, around when kids first start to develop an interest in the passage to adulthood and continuing into their college or early work years when social pressure makes the holding and handling of cigarettes highly desirable.

To be truly effective, the health movement has to offer a powerful and socially desirable reward system. It also has to affect smokers at a very personal level; it needs to provide a vehicle for them to find their mythic role in life and face the key challenges that define the value of their existence. It seems ridiculous that tobacco companies have actually fallen into a business that offers just such a product. But, as any marketer knows, it is not *how* smart you or your product is, it is how strong is the need you are able to fill. The psychic need these products fulfill along with the inability of an advanced, rational society to deliver a positive alternative to them has left a huge gap. Is it any wonder that it has been filled by a legion of lowlifes from corner drug dealers to tobacco merchants, and in, some cases, even seemingly responsible pharmaceutical manufacturers?

The Vision Quest movement would need the support of counselors, teachers, and industry to develop a vast, yet personalized network of trainers, mentors, and a reward system to help people manage this passage through life. But the essential idea of using existing activity systems, but adding a reward, certification, and a new dimension of meaning in societal status is probably the most practical.

Sports, games, videogame tournaments for the serious, hiking, boating or even dance efforts can be harnessed to deliver the program. Anyone who participates in these activities can ask to be rated as a participant on a smoke avoidance Vision Quest plan. They are then brought into a network of mentors and counselors who help them find their Vision Quest role in the activity. As they progress, they are rated and rewarded on the basis of their relationship to others in the program, as a separate reward system from that which occurs in the game itself. With community and commercial support, participants will be offered rewards from health-conscious catalog items to planned trips, camps, scholarships, public exposure, job preferences, and a number of rewards that society in general can offer.

At its bare bones level, this would be like taking the pledge in return for points in a book of awards. This system must also have a way to offer and manage the teens' need for a Vision Quest. That is the critical difference between this and, for example, a DARE campaign which does some of these things, but offers teens little more than "just say no" when it comes to fulfilling their specific psychic and social needs.

The other difference between a Vision Quest system and boy scout rating system is that this system is not necessarily hierarchical. It can be. But the point is really about helping young people to find their identity. So the key part of the quest is that find a role and a title: a specialty or key skill that identifies that young person, one that signifies acceptance and then status.

The exploitation of the Vision Quest issue can even be seen in the development of suicide bombers. The mythic quest of Islam coupled with a reward system both on earth and in the afterlife has enabled radical Islamic and other terror groups to produce a steady group of recruits. It could be argued that smokers are a slow motion version of the same phenomenon but without the desire to harm others.

Imagine the real internal dialog of a susceptible teen: "I want to go to college and perhaps become a lawyer but I'm not sure. And I want to look stronger/prettier and I want to be able deal better with peers and members of the opposite sex. I want to be inspired somehow. I want to feel like I have accomplished something. I want to feel important. I want to create my own path." Let's add a dash of Campbell: "I want to follow my bliss....."

Does anything we have now address these issues?

In a typical society we can offer a formal education and a little school counseling but none of that gets at the big question of who you are, why are you on this on this earth, and what will your chosen profession do to nurture your soul? Myths deal with this and the tobacco pseudo-myths offer a very simple means to accomplish this sensation. Even at two or three times the 1987 price, cigarettes are still an inexpensive solution compared to the costs college, pharmaceuticals, and a feeling of being stranded. All we really offer now is sports, but that only affects the few who have real sporting talent; everyone else is left out. Besides, not all sports present a Vision Quest solution. Sports can be dangerously competitive in a number of ways that are destructive or may encourage cheating and irresponsible behavior, thanks to the special indulgence society grants to alpha leaders and other types of conquerors. Also, sports are a relatively fixed universe: football, baseball, basketball, and a handful of other games. The human psyche demands a much richer playing field.

That vast social/personal identity gap is the one where society has to manufacture a healthy solution or the old tobacco and drug solutions will continue to take their toll. Indeed, they continue to do so anyway but they do it in a way that is unchallenged at the level that really counts – in their relevance to the teens themselves. In other words, it is all very well to say that smoking and, for that matter, all kinds of drug using is bad. And you can lock up the worst abusers and the dealers who break the law. But if the motivation for smoking is not somehow quenched, the simple equation remains unchanged: people on a Vision Quest, no matter how dangerous, are impervious to reason. So, fighting the quest without addressing the issue of motivation simply causes an escalation of the negative results we have already encountered in the drug-use world: rapid growth in the jailing of users but no drop in overall drug use.

A similar fate awaits smoking if the public health groups rely on opprobrium and the recitation of health warnings as their only weapons.

Let us imagine for one minute that the health movement ran a Hollywood studio. The movement would feel compelled to issue a warning with every car chase, stating that this is dangerous behavior and statistically it is better to let the criminals get away because they are likely to get caught over time, and that no property or physical damage is worth the risk of the chase. Likewise, if health professionals were commissioned with rewriting Homer's Odyssey it might warn Ulysses that warfare is a dangerous activity or they might tell Jason that seeking a Golden Fleece without a proper map and in a dangerous, unknown place is foolhardy and not worth the risk. It might show there is a distinct lack of evidence that the golden fleece actually exists and scientists doubt that such a thing, even if it existed, could live up to any of its claims.

In other words, the health movement has the benefit of being right but lacks the ability to address the great quests of the unconscious, which are eternal, uncaring of danger, and ever-listening to the sound of what seems to be a higher, or more soulful calling.

Until we talk to the teens on that level and address those issues, we really are not talking to them at all. Even when I was growing up and tobacco was still in its glory days, 11 year old kids seemed to know a great deal about the dangers of smoking. "It'll kill ya," were the actual words of my 11 year old friend who unveiled a bunch of half smoked butts he stole from his father's ashtray. He went on to talk about how it damaged the lungs. But the mystery of why his Dad and so many people did it anyway was too much for him and we both had to try it. We coughed, we were disgusted, and in my case I remember actively criticizing my father for being a smoker. I was dead against it. I should have been a poster boy for the anti-smoking movement – and most children probably are. But I became a smoker anyway and so will many others who seemed at one time to be against it. That is because they have no idea what of life's crossroads they will come upon as they reach their teen years.

Even in my college years, the most fervent smoker I knew was also the most knowledgeable about the damage to his lungs. A fine discussion for him began with a description of the killing of the lung's cilia. Knowledge is in and of itself not the answer; it is just the beginning. The real answer lies in the Vision Quest issue.

This book, too, is the product of a kind of Vision Quest. Its moment of origin in the late nineteen seventies came with the insight that **Marlboro** was a "medal." With that knowledge, I began a strange journey, first as a fledgling adman. Then, as the idea grew to encompass the initiation concept as embodied in its original tattoo campaign, it began to really bother the creative directors I sought to work for. I never got the job of selling cigarettes that I reluctantly pursued. When I saw that the ideas I **took** around were being pilfered, I was driven to take this injustice and turn it into a true understanding of the apparent language of smoking and the mysteries of the coming-of-age ritual. It never bothered me that so few people from academia to publishers were willing to give the theories any credence whatsoever. I believed I had broken an important code. When Google's pay-per-click advertising emerged on the internet, I found a low-cost way to attract hundreds of smokers from the U.S, Canada, and the U.K. to fill out questionnaires to provide an empirical basis for these theories. Now, a growing body of MRI research on the brain adds its support to the nature and profundity of the smoking experience. While I continued to finance the project myself without public backers, save a few hardy souls like John Leo of U.S News who had tilted his own lance at the tobacco windmills, the journey, as in all Vision Quests, brought its own reward. Thanks to John, I was introduced to my true intellectual mentor, Ernest Dichter, with whom I spent time in the last two years of his life and at whose memorial I spoke. It would also be hard not to thank Joseph Campbell – although you have no idea how hard it is to show people how the activities of exotic primitives in obscure places is being replicated in their own back yards – in a disguised form!

Somehow, this journey took me into the computer business, arguably the most unlikely place for a neo-mythicist. The combination of graphics and word processing led me there and, once employed in the business, I made a fine living. Yet, I never gave up on the idea and simply waited for its time, evolving each part of this extraordinary insight. I remember being inspired by the plight of Nelson Mandela, whom I first heard of as boy when I saw signs on railroad bridges and other inaccessible places proclaiming, "Free Nelson Mandela." At the time, I thought," Why not?" When I asked my parents who Nelson Mandela was, they replied "sssshhhhh." And so I always felt that if he could wait so long – and in jail - for freedom, why couldn't I wait in the pleasures of the free world for this idea's time to come?

I would like to think that all teens have their own personal vision that, once found, has its own means of sustenance, to give their lives meaning and that can carry them through their worldly existence. The point about a Vision Quest is that even if you don't come back with the golden fleece, the journey takes you to the places that sustain you and give your life meaning.

The problem is that most teens have no idea how to find their vision, and the official world they live in gives them precious little assistance in finding it. So, they are forced into the underworld and the false habits of the commercial marketplace which always expands to fill a need. The marketplace has no responsibility to fulfill the needs properly and may not even know why it is there, other than that it is responding to a profitable market opportunity.

Becoming a guide in the Vision Quest of teenagers may be a lot more than anyone who took on the smoking issue bargained for, but it is vital in order to maintain relevancy. More to the point, the concerned public health groups will continue to get precious little of the settlement money unless they step up to the plate with a plan.

We have the rare experience in life to take on hundreds of years of misguided behavior and suddenly reorder it in a way that makes great sense for humanity. This is our moment in time. Let us hope we can seize it.

WHY E-CIGARETTES WILL CHANGE EVERYTHING.

It is appropriate, given the slightly mystical approach of this book, that the most significant development in the world of smoking since the invention of the cellulose filter in the 1950's or the great US tobacco settle in 1997 began as a dream.

Hon Lik was a chemist in China suffering from early stage emphysema and watching his father die of lung cancer from smoking. Just as the discovery of the double helix structure of DNA came to James Watson as a symbolic dream of two intertwined snakes, so Hon had a dream of his own. According to the story in the L.A. Times in April 2009, "Hon says the idea of the electronic cigarettes came to him in a dream in 2000: Coughing and wheezing, he imagined he was drowning, until suddenly the waters around him lifted into a fog."

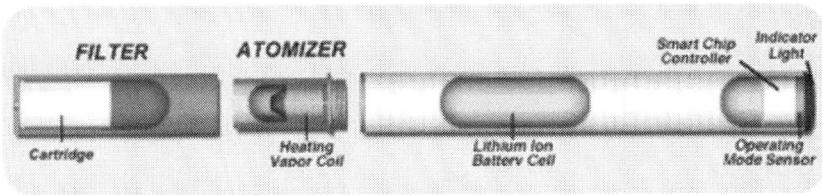

Since then, Shenzen, China has become the heart of this new kind of cigarette manufacturing industry - a minor masterpiece of microelectronic technology and chemical reconstitution. Instead of lighting up the traditional dried and processed tobacco leaves, you puff on a something that looks like a cigarette but is as solid as a pen. When you puff, a tiny sensor notices the pressure and sets a miniature vaporizer to life. The vaporizer taps a small container of nicotine and flavorings suspended in propylene glycol or some other natural liquid. Voila! a steady stream of nicotine-delivering vapor comes your way and you are freed from an odious trip to the outhouse and arguably, an array of health issues that accompany it.

The magic is in the sensor, the tiny vaporizer and the marvel of rechargeable ni-cad batteries. To the vaper, they now have an acceptable "smoke". No smell, no second-hand smoke and no cancer-inducing tar. The jury is still out on whether propylene glycol – an inert liquid used in aerosols and dozens of other household products, is itself dangerous. So far there are no studies proving their danger or safety – even after nearly 10 years on the market.

While there is some controversy over propylene glycol he product is on the FDA's Generally Accepted as Safe list. Still, there are numerous medical people who say otherwise. They may well have an agenda of their own – usually tied to anti-smoking funding or a sense of their own self-righteousness. In any case, the odds are, by the time the data comes in, we will have moved onto some other vaping medium. What matters is that smoking has begun its inexorable journey of change.

It is a good guess that efforts by the FDA and various municipalities to ban e-Cigs will backfire. The two main reasons are that e-Cigs are not exactly catching fire right now, so the moment it becomes seen as a rebellious product, it will gain in stature – or as we like to say – in spirit power. The other reason is that the politics behind their opposition are becoming increasingly apparent and they usually have an ulterior motive.

At the same time, a major attraction of e-Cigarettes are their lack of "second-hand smoke" damage and vaping is almost bother-free to others in the room. There is simply a mist but no actual smell. So vapers will get the typical tobacco smell off their clothes, cars, homes and offices (if they are allowed back in!). Their breaths will return to sweetness, discoloration will vanish from their teeth and fingers and their lungs may even have a chance to resuscitate. They will also save enough on their regular habit – depending on their local taxation – to make the monthly payments on a Honda Accord or a Ford Fiesta.

Oddly, e-Cigarettes have not taken off anywhere nearly as much as you'd think. In 2009 there were an estimated 500,000 e-Cigarette smokers in the US out of a population of around 40 million cigarette smokers.

There are a number of - reasons some of them obvious and some that require furious head scratching. The price barrier for e-Cigarettes ranges from around $70 and up to a few hundred dollars for the reusable kits and as low as $10 and less for the disposables.

E-Cigarettes are not available in many retail outlets – they are mostly sold online. Thanks to spammers and the lack of recognizable brands there is a strong element of consumer distrust. Many producers lock the "vapers" into their own brand of replaceable flavorant and nicotine supplies – sometimes known as "drip." The savvy or adventurous know they can buy this online from many sources. The overall market seems confusing and in disarray.

Then there are scare stories from anti-cancer groups and certain doctors. While it is true that no studies have shown that e-Cigarettes are safe, there are also no studies that show they aren't. So it is odd that so many public-spirited groups are indirectly supporting a product that is known to be deadly because the replacement *isn't known to be deadly*. They have a right to be cautious but when you peel back the covers you generally find these groups are in a symbiotic relationship with the tobacco companies. They are often being funded by tobacco settlement money and taxes on smoking.

The biggest problem is that real smokers think e-Cigarettes are pale imitations of the real thing. In other words, they kind of suck.

To that we can only say, if you understand what your brand gives you psychologically then you can learn to shift it to your e-Cigarette and from there, to any medium that you choose.

Like any revolution, there are a zillion reasons why things won't change in the tobacco world. Luckily, revolutions happen because they must. You can't herd 40 million people onto the street in the middle of winter or treat them like lepers forever. Something has to give and smokers will find a way to rebel or someone will sell them on a tool that brings them back to the regular world.

E-Cigarettes are clearly the opening in the dam – they unquestionably hold the key to the next generation of "spirit" ingestion. The prices will fall away – indeed, if you bought this book directly, you were entitled to a free deposable e-Cig. So if this book can do it many others will follow.

The medical issues will be overcome – at least in the sense that some form of vapor will wind up being much safer on the lungs than any form of smoke. For all we know, someone might invent a benign smoke in the future. What matters is that innovation is taking place in a way that has never happened before.

As smokers become energized by the possibility that they are not entirely mad and they can rejoin normal life thanks to e-Cigarettes, we may enter a different culture. When society understands that smoking is really a non-pharmaceutical way of maintaining psychic balance then they will think very differently about e-Cigarettes. They may be less judgmental than they are on their Prozac- and Valium-taking friends.

So let's understand what they e-Cigarettes really are. Technically, they are a slick but simple device for ingesting flavored nicotine. It is rigid where cigarettes are firm but tender. They are pristine and their fumes feel like breaths in winter – but without the iciness – something like a visit to an ice rink or the fog machine at a flashy disco.

Smokers are giving up two of the most important elements of smoke – the delicious, earthy, sensuousness of actual tobacco and the invasion of the lungs by a mild intoxicant. Even though most cigarettes are really chemically enhanced reconstituted tobacco bits, they still have more reality than e-Cigarettes' "techno haze." Gone too is the deep unconscious connection to a loving mommy and her special body odor that tobacco companies and their fake fragrance suppliers have long ago mastered and slipped into the tube. Gone is the tenderness of a smoky trail or a long drag of comfort.

Given the pharma-tobacco trade-off, it is very likely that vaping might wind up being a platform for many kinds of ingestions. We already see Viagra and THC being slipped into some willing vapers e-Cigs. That may be the biggest fear of the political and moral establishment. How do you control it? Perhaps just as importantly, how do you tax it?

Politicians will probably figure out a way. Let's rather understand what it means to smokers.

If you want to quit, e-Cigarettes can be a great first step, precisely because they force you to give up those two critical elements in smoking – the attachment to eternal, maternal comfort and the ingestion of spirit power through acrid smoke. So, if you can overcome those two elements you're on your way to quitting forever and here is how:

Let's says you find a couple of substiitutes to carry you over the great chasm of quitting cigarettes. Say you begin by combining gum and e-Cigs. At some point you can dump the cigarettes and now you are half way to quitting the psychological part. All you have to do is roll back the smoking years and deal with the issues you faced at initiation.

Then you take on an alternate ritual that covers what you *would* have done if you *hadn't* smoked, and voila you are on your way. Along this journey you could alternate between regular and e-Cig smoking but sooner or later, you are going to have to choose one over the other. So, assuming you have the ability to go forward with e-Cigs, then you are ready to handle the next big step. You can even begin doing this before you have completely given up regular cigarettes. In fact you should start doing this right now, in easy careful steps.

At that point, you face the inevitable issue, what if you can't give up e-Cigs? The answer is, if you believe the word of many other e-smokers, you can give up e-Cigs any time – it is much easier than regular cigarettes. Of course, regular smokers say that too and we have all learned not to believe them. But with e-Cigs, they might be telling the truth. These things *are* a little cold, so maybe people *can* really quit at will. In that case, vaping may just be too convenient and inexpensive for them to not keep on doing it – at least for a while.

That may be a big concern for the medical profession. You can vape or not, at will. It becomes an interesting platform for other kinds of mind- and performance-altering substances that have come to dominate our lives since these can deliver to the lungs which is the body's quickest point of absorption. Sure, you could always pop a pill but there might be some substances that are worth vaping.

If you have anxiety pangs in a social setting, a vapor laced with Zoloft might not be such a bad idea. Our media friends who once chainsmoked through deadlines nd have moved on to DD medications might prefer to vape their

Ridalin, and enjoy the companionship of an e-Cig rather than the coldness of a pill with water.

My favorite future possible use is on people with dangerous dispositions - like potential serial killers who are at risk of going off their meds. Combing their antidepressants with a nicotine laced e-Cig may not be such a bad idea. They might not shoot anyone if they remain on their pills. Of course, nicotine may not be the best addictant but someone will inevitably perfect just the right chemical for the job – of keeping at-risk people on their medications. Keeping potential killers and sex offenders on their meds just may be another reason why the e-Cig is really a platform for new kinds of self-medication.

So why not? The fact that e-Cigs are hard to get in retail environments will soon change. One way or another hey will become ubiquitous and the question will be: did we get left behind? Has our troubled relationship with America's first industry left us in the lurch as once more, China takes the lead?

MAKING CIGARETTE SEMIOTICS WORK FOR YOU
THE BRAND PERSONALITY PROFILE

What We Look For

Most smokers start with the cigarettes that are around them. If family members smoke, sooner or later smokers will try their band. They may try on a number of bands. So what we look for are the brands smokers experimented with and just who introduced them. If their parents smoked, it is critical to know what brands. Once the smoker settles on the brand we can draw picture of who that person is; in handwriting analysis, that would be like finding the gestalt. From then, on we can interpret the meaning of each brand these smokers take on or avoid, as they go through life.

Generally, smokers experiment with a number of brands before they settle in on their main brand. We also ask about alternative brands, the ones they will smoke if they can't get their regular brand. Then, just as important, we ask what brands they won't smoke – these are their taboo brands.

As smokers move through life, they can change their brands. But they rarely do it without reason. The brands could reflect a gradual change in smokers' personality but often they reflect an abrupt change in their life situation. In fact, if there is no change in brand profile over a lifetime, then you have a very stagnant personality.

The most common change is the coming of middle age. Based on our three country profiles (U.S, U.K, and Canada) this seems to occur at around age 40.

At that age, men will tend to face up to the long term danger of smoking and make their adjustments. Typically, they will step down to a lower-tar version of their original smoke. So, **Marlboro** regular will come out as **Marlboro** Mild or **Marlboro** Light.

Often though, the male smoker will move to a brand that honors an historic connection to smoking or introduces some type of philosophical statement. So, middle age men in the U.S might adopt American Spirit as a way of honoring the Native American ritual of smoking. In the U.K., male smokers often turn to hand-rolling their own with something like the brand Old Holborn.

Women, especially in the lower classes, will often turn to ultra-feminine brands like Eve or Misty as away to hang onto their youthful sexuality. Typically, they will select a long version as a reflection of their yearning or resistance to change.

How Brand Attachments are Formed

The underlying theory **of** the meanings of the individual brands also enables **us** to apply a kind of "grammar" to brands. Using anecdotal insight, **we** can discover a way to look at the personality of the smokers behind the brands. There are stages of a smoker's life **as he or she** go through a number of recognizable changes**,** and this is reflected in their brand switching, which helps when **we make** an analysis. While the smoking symbols are relatively simple, the smokers are not. So we look at the brands as merely their point of contact with the greater force in life. Like a biblical character, it tells **us** what they will sacrifice before Jehovah and why. **Smokers** are fully aware of the dangers**,** at least at some level and they yearn, past all measure of reasonableness, for a higher intervention. Moreover, they are willing to participate in *cultus deus*, the act of "caring for the god**,**" by taking on addiction and making communion every twenty minutes or so with a smoke. Great **and small** people alike have been smokers. That is not to diminish humanity**;** it is simply to say that the divine power we have been willing to assign it is just that much greater than any kind of human.

The secret then, is in the power we have been willing to assign it – and in many, many cases, the lack of an alternative. We want God, we want myth and we want ritual in our life. We just need to know what it is, **and** how it works**,** and **then how to** go find a better source.

How This Book Came to be Written

This book came to be written because of a campaign this author produced for a then imaginary brand of cigarettes called Benson's in 1980. The campaign was based on a unique analysis of the **Marlboro** Man story and what was, in effect, an early prototype of the semiotic theory employed in this book.

When the campaign emerged in the form of a new brand called Barclay, produced by the McCann-Erickson agency, it became clear that the underlying subject was deserving of deeper examination. This resulted in a paper presented in 1984 at the Annual Convention of the Popular Culture Society, produced by Bowling Green University, Ohio in Toronto and has resulted in this book, **Cigarette Seduction.**

Biographical Notes

This book came about because of this author's interest **back in the nineteen seventies** in the way information is transmitted, a dissatisfaction with the efficiency of the written word, and a subsequent search to find a new, visually-based method of communication. The result is a kind of "street semiotic" and a unique model for understanding the practice of smoking.

The odyssey began at Columbia University where **my** strong interest in the meaning of art grew into a quest that followed this unusual path. **My quest started with** a long visit to England and a fascination with the revolution that was taking place in the ad industry there. Many new ideas were taking shape and the differences between ad communication in the **U.K.** and the **U.S.** provided nuggets of fascinating information about symbolic expression. Madison Avenue seemed like the ideal place to develop and launch **this** idea since it was in the business of probing the visual consciousness of the public and offering up a constantly changing symbolic language.

However, in order **for me** to get into Madison Avenue it was necessary to produce advertising. As a two-pack-a-day smoker at the time and sufficiently interested in making a good living without worrying overly about the consequences, I chose to handle products that were worthy of attention. Having spent **my** formative years in Africa, I had also been fascinated by the fact that American brands succeeded in appealing to dissimilar cultures throughout the world. Camel, **Kent,** and **Marlboro** were the leading examples. Yet, somehow, **Marlboro** stood out from among them all.

In 1980, when I moved to New York, I produced what is commonly known among copywriters as a "book" or portfolio of samples. As a smoker and someone who knew **his** way around the whiskies of Scotland, I produced an ad campaign for a new kind of cigarette along with a series of ads for a pure malt whisky. Then I threw in a new campaign for Coca-Cola. I also began a study of the **Marlboro** story, where I learned about its dress change and first saw the famous tattoo ad. I began then to recognize that a certain anthropological custom I had seen before in Africa was being played out on the billboards and magazines of America.

As this advertising "book" was being developed and taken around to various agencies it attracted the attention of a few good ad men. It went to Art Einstein when he was the copy chief at Lord Geller Federico & Einstein. He scoffed at **the "book,"** but one of his art directors, Seymon Ostilly, helped to clean it up and bring it into focus. In particular, he and an old copywriter friend of his, Milt Trazenfeld, helped with the Coke campaign, "Wherever you go. Coke is..." and then he did the illustrations on the campaign for a single malt whisky called Laphroiag: "**It's whispered in high places.**"

By the time I reached Scali, McCabe & Sloves to see Larry Cadman, a creative director, my research on the **Marlboro** Man had born fruit in the campaign for a new, imaginary brand of cigarettes called Bensons, an obvious play on the Philip Morris brand, Benson & Hedges. Cadman looked at this campaign for an imagined brand of cigarettes - the one with the James Bond-like character and a woman looking over his shoulder - and commented on the suit and tie he was wearing. "Make that a tuxedo." He also suggested I get rid of the scar on his face. I took his advice on the tuxedo but resisted him on the scar. I knew the **Marlboro** Man had an initiation mark and I wanted something similar for mine, which is why I chose an alternate to a tattoo - a cicatrix.

Finally, I took this book to McCann-Erickson, the agency of record for Coca-Cola and to Brown & Williamson (then working on an about-to-be-announced brand of cigarettes called Barclay). The book stayed at McCann's for less than a week and the personnel manager I spoke to who said she had sent it on to the creative director, Scott Miller, returned it without comment.

Within a year, Coca-Cola had abandoned their "Have a Coke and a Smile" campaign for a new one McCann-Erickson claims to have devised that went: "Coke is it." My original thesis for dropping the smile campaign was based on the inspiration I had received from a defaced subway poster; someone had blacked out one of the teeth of a smiling Coke drinker. I argued **that, obviously,** if you talk about smiling, and colas have a reputation for being bad for the teeth, then it is only a matter of time before **this** backfires at some level of consciousness. Somebody at McCann-Erickson must have agreed with that and dropped their campaign for **one that was** arguably mine.

Then Barclay came out with the slogan "99% Tar Free," which is not something to which I make any claim. However, the Barclay man himself was the same James Bond-like character that I had presented with a tuxedo and, instead of the scar, a dimple and the trademark **female** glancing over his shoulder. After that, some McCann refugees **moved** to a new agency called Backer & Spielvogel (now Backer Spielvogel Bates) where they initiated a campaign for a whisky that went, "J&B. It whispers."

It had been my intention to create a new kind of archetype and they had obviously recognized that from my "book" but chose not to give me any credit for it. That is not unusual among creative enterprises that are as highly competitive as advertising. While it not possible to condone the essential dishonesty of these agencies, the real point of the "book" was to describe the symbolic process rather than just the ability to produce a few good ads. Once it became clear that. for reasons of originality, it was unlikely that the process, as embodied in that "book" would ever find real acceptance in an ad agency, it seemed reasonable to apply that knowledge to the subject at hand and examine the mythos of smoking. After all, it was out of a mythic journey into the Western psyche that I had conceived these ideas in the first place. So, finding the time, I took courses at the New School where this book began to be formulated.

After a varied journey as **an** inventor, a computer marketer, **and a** technology marketing journalist with such publications as **ADWEEK's Marketing Computers**, **Advertising Age Creativity**, **MacWEEK**, **this** author is now president of TECHmarketing, a specialty conference company that produces conferences and capital-raising forums for New Media companies.

Why eCigarettes Will Change Everything

It is appropriate, given the slightly mystical approach of this book, that the most significant development in the world of smoking since the invention of the cellulose filter in the 1950's began as a dream.

Hon Lik was a chemist in China suffering from early stage emphysema and watching his father die of lung cancer from smoking. Just as the discovery of the double helix structure of DNA came to James Watson as a symbolic dream of two intertwined snakes, so Hon had a dream of his own. According to the story in the L.A. Times in April 2009, "Hon says the idea of the electronic cigarettes came to him in a dream in 2000: Coughing and wheezing, he imagined he was drowning, until suddenly the waters around him lifted into a fog."

Since then, Shenzen, China has become the heart of this new kind of cigarette manufacturing industry - a minor masterpiece of microelectronic technology and chemical reconstitution. Instead of lighting up the traditional dried and processed tobacco leaves, you puff on a something that looks like a cigarette but is as solid as a pen. When you puff, a tiny sensor notices the pressure and sets a miniature vaporizer to life. The vaporizer taps a small container of nicotine and flavorings suspended in propylene glycol or a some other natural liquid. Voila! a steady stream of nicotine deliver vapor comes your way and you are freed from, smell a trip to the outhouse and arguably, health issues.

The magic is in the sensor, the tiny vaporizer and the magic of rechargeable ni-cad batteries. To the vaper, they now have an acceptable "smoke". No smell, no second-hand smoke and no cancer-inducing tar. The jury is still out on whether propylene glycol – an inert liquid used in aerosols and dozens of other household products, are themselves dangerous. So far there are no studies proving their danger or safety – even after nearly 10 years on the market.

While there is come controversy over propylene glycol which is on the FDA's list of Generally Accepted as Safe list, there are numerous medical people who say otherwise. They may well have an agenda of their own – usually tied to anti-smoking funding or a sense of their own self-righteousness. In any case, the odds are, by the time the data comes in, we will have moved onto some other vaping medium. What matters is that smoking has begun its inexorable journey of change.

It is a good guess that efforts by the FDA and various municipalities to ban e-Cigs will backfire. The two main reasons are that they are not exactly catching fire right now, so the moment it becomes seen as a rebellious product it will gain in stature – or as we like to say – in spirit power. The other reason is the that the politics of their opposition are becoming increasingly apparent

Whatever, we think of the "second-hand" damage this is barely an issue with vaping. So vapers will get the smell off their clothes, cars, homes and offices (if they are allowed back in!). Their breaths will return to sweetness, discoloring will vanish form their teeth and fingers and lungs may have a chance to resuscitate. They will also save enough on their regular habit – depending on where you live – to make the monthly payments on a Honda Accord or a Ford Fiesta.

Oddly, these products have not taken off anywhere nearly as much as you'd think. In 2009 there were an estimated 500,000 e-Cigarette smokers in the US out of a population of around 40 million.

There are a number of - reasons some of them obvious and some that require furious head scratching. The price barrier for these products is quite high starting at around $70 and up to a few hundred dollars for the reusable kits and as low as around $10 for the disposables.

They are not available in may retail outlets – its mostly online.

There are scare stories from anti-cancer groups and certain doctors.

Real smokers think these products are pale imitations of the real thing. In other words, they kind of suck.

Like any revolution, there are a zillion reasons why things won't change. Luckily revolutions happen because they must. You can't herd 40 million people onto the street in the middle of winter or treat them like lepers forever. Something has to give, smokers will find a way to rebel or someone sells them a tool that brings them back to the regular world.

E-Cigarettes are clearly the opening in the dam – they unquestionable hold the key to the next generation of spirit ingestion. The prices will fall away. If you bought this book, you were entailed to free deposable E-Cig and in many ways other swill follow.

The medical issues will be overcome – at least in the sense that some form of vaper will wind up being much safer on the lungs than any form of smoke. Although, who know someone might invent a benign smoke in the future. What mattes is that innovation is taking place in an entirely new area.

As smokers become energized by the possibility that they are not entirely mad and they can rejoin normal like – in fact converts might ween oin thme , they will think very differently about e-Cigarettes.

So let's understand what they really are. Technically, it's a slick but simple device for ingesting flavored nicotine. It is rigid where cigarettes are firm but tender. Its pristine fumes feels like breaths in winter – but without the iciness. A visit to an ice rink or the fog machine at a flashy disco.

Smokes are giving two of the most important elements of smoke – the delicious, earthy, sensuousness of actual tobacco. Vent chemical enhanced reconstirgued tobacco bits have more reality than this techno haze. Gone is the connection to a loving mommy and her special body odor. Gone is the tenderness of a smoke or a long drag of comfort.

Actually, the vapers might wind up being a platform for many kinds of ingestions. That is probably the biggest fear of the political establishment. How do you control it? Perhaps just as importantly, how do you tax it?

Politicians will probably figure out a way. Let's rather understand what it means to smokers.

If you want to quit, e-Cigarettes can be a great first step, precisely because they force you to give up those two critical elements in smoking – the attachment to eternal, maternal comfort. So, if you can overcome those two elements. Lets says you find a couple of substiitutes to carry you over. Say, gum and e-Cigs then at some point you can dump the cigarettes and now you are half way to quitting the psychological part. All you have to do is roll back the smoking years and deal with the issues you faced at initaitination.

Take on a alternate ritual that covers what you *would* have done if you *hadn't* smoked, and voila you are on your way. Along the way you could alternate between regular and e-Cig smoking but sooner or later, you are going to have to choose one over the others. So, assuming you have the ability to go forward with e-Cigs you are ready to handle the next big step. You can even begin doing this before you have completely given up regulars, in fact you should start doing this right now, in easy careful steps.

At that point, you face the inevitable issue, what if you cant give up e-Cigs? The answer, if you believe them, is that you can give up e-Cigs any times – it is much easier than regular cigarettes. Of course, regular smokers say that too but we have all learned not to believe them. Bu with e-Cigs, they might be telling the truth. These things *are* a little cold, so maybe people *can* really quit at will. In that case, vaping may just be too convenient and inexpensive for them to not keep on doing it – at least for a while.

That may be a big concern for the medical profession but it becomes an interesting platform for other kinds of mind an performance altering substances that have come to dominate our lives. Sure you could pop a pill but there might be some substances that are worth vaping.

If you have anxiety pangs in a social setting, a vaper laced with Zoloft might not be such a bad idea. Our media friends on dealing might prefer to vapor their ridalin, and enjoy the companionship of an eCig rather than the coldness of a pill with water.

My favorite is people with dangerous dispositions, like potential serial killers who have a habit of going off their meds. Combing their antidepressants with a nicotine laced e_Cig may not be such a bad idea.

They might not have shot anyone had they been on the pill. Of course nicotine may not be the best addictant but someone will inenivitably perfect just the right chemical for the job. Another reason why the e-Cig is really a platform for new kinds of self-medication.

So why not? The fact that e-Cigs are hard to get in retail environments will soon change. One way or another hey will become ubiquitous and the question will be: did we get left behind?

TECHNICAL BIBLIOGRAPHY:

Art and Visual Perception……..……....Rudolph Arnheim, U. Cal., 1974
Ashes to Ashes…………………………Richard Kluger, Random House, 1996
Basis for Marketing Decision……...........Louis Cheskin, Liveright, 1961
Biography of an Idea…………………………E.L. Bernays, S&S, 1965
Cigarette Country……………………..………Susan Wagner, Praeger, 1971
Cigarettes Are Sublime……Richard Klein, Duke University Press, 1995
The Cigarette Papers…..……Stanton A. Glantz, California U. Press, 1995
Coming of Age in Samoa………………Margaret Mead, Morrow, 1928
Confessions of an Advertising Man…..….David Ogilvy, Atheneum, 1963
Decoding Advertisements……….……Judith Williamson, Boyars, 1978
Diagrams of the Unconscious…..Werner Wolff, Grune & Stratton, 1948
Dictionary of Trade Name Origins……….Adrian Room, Routledge Kegan Paul, 1982
Growing up in New Guinea……………Margaret Mead, Morrow, 1930
Handbook of Consumer Motivations…Ernest Dichter, McGraw-Hill, '64
Handbook of Package Design Research……….Walter Stern, Wiley, 1981
How to Predict What People Will Buy..Louis Cheskin, Liveright, 1957
Icons of America……………Browne & Fishwick, Popular Press, 1978
Industrial Design……………………Raymond Loewy, Overlook, 1979
Madison Avenue, USA……………Martin Meyer, McGraw-Hill, 1991
Motivating Human Behavior………..Ernest Dichter, McGraw-Hill, 1971
Motivation in Advertising……..…Pierre Martineau, McGraw-Hill, 1957
Objects of Special Devotion……………Ray B. Browne, Popular Press,
Ogilvy on Advertising…………………………David Ogilvy, Crown, 1983
Packaging Power………………………Walter Margulies, World, 1970
Packaging -- The Sixth Sense?……………Ernest Dichter, Cahners, 1975
Positioning: The Battle for Your Mind…………Ries & Trout, McGraw-Hill, 1981
Preconscious Processing………………...…Norman Dixon, Wiley, 1981
Reality in Advertising……………...………Rosser Reeves, Knopf, 1961
Marketing Management……………Joseph W. Newman, Harvard, 1957
Scientific Advertising……………Claude Hopkins, Lord & Thomas, 1923
Smokescreen…………………………Phillip J. Hilts, Addison-Wesley 1996
Secrets of Marketing Success……………Louis Cheskin, Trident, 1967
Studies in Expressive Movement….Allport & Vernon, Macmillan, 1933
Tested Advertising Methods………John Caples, Prentice-Hall, 1974
The 100 Greatest Advertisements…………Julian Watkins, Dover, 1959
The Engineering of Consent……………E.L. Bernays, U. Okla., 1955
The Mirror Makers…………………………Stephen Fox, Morrow, 1984
The Naked Ape…………………Desmond Morris, McGraw-Hill, 1967

The Rage to Persuade..........................Bleustein-Blanchet, Chelsea, 1982

The Search for Oneness........Silverman Lachman & Milich, International U., 1982

The Sexual Lives of Savages........Bronislaw Malinowski, Halcyon, 1929

The Strategy of Desire...........................Ernest Dichter, Doubleday, 1960

The Tobacco Problem.........................Meta Lander, De Wolfe Fisk, 1885

The Trouble With Advertising..........John O'Toole, Chelsea House, 1981

They Satisfy......................................Robert Sobel, Anchor, 1978

Understanding Consumer Behavior.......M. Grossack, Christopher, 1964

Why People Buy....................................Louis Cheskin, Liveright, 1959

BOOKS & ARTICLES OF RELATED INTEREST:

Warning: nicotine seriously improves health.........Guardian: Sunday July 18, 2004

www.guardian.co.uk/smoking/Story/0,2763,1263918,00.html

Body Language... **Jules Fast, Pocket, 1971**
The first popular book on reading character from people's non-verbal clues. Very "pop" and lacking a central theory, both on why we give out these signals and how to systematically interpret them.

Cigarette Seduction explains why the external signals reflect the states of our inner selves and describes a simple but profound interpretive method. Body language is old hat now but cigarette symbolism has never been touched.

Cigarette Pack Art... **Chris Mullen, St. Martin's, 1979**
The first book to elaborate **on** the visually symbolic world of cigarette packaging. Makes no attempt to infer either why people smoke or what the brands tell us about the smoker. Coffee table/Art Director's book.

Cigarette Seduction takes the messages on the packs and in the advertising and explains everything. Everything.

Hero With a Thousand Faces .... **Joseph   Campbell, Princeton, 1949**
No question, Joe Campbell made people understand that mythologies are not fairy tales but moral tales that help us decide how to deal with our journey through life. But Campbell's books only work well when the reader transports himself to another culture; **t**hey are strangely lacking when it comes to telling us how a white collar worker in Kansas may uncover **his** "hero's journey." Cigarettes happen to be a modern if controversial way of exploring this path.

The best Campbell can say is "follow your bliss." That is a little like saying you get from Greenwich Village to 110th St. by going up 7th Avenue **but** neglecting to say that you have to watch out for Times Square or that Central Park is in the way so that the normal road disappears and you can't go at night. With cigarettes and **Cigarette Seduction** we find that people have discovered an informal answer to the hero's journey - complete with road signs, power symbols, and a penetrating view of the soul as it reaches for, say, a Camel.

The Hidden Persuaders .... Vance   Packard,   McKay **1957**

The first! This is the perennially popular book that first exposed Madison Avenue as the true temple of psychology in America. It has shocked and titillated people ever since its beginnings as a mere article by a journalist. Not only are its insights truer than ever but they are the common baggage -- knowingly and unknowingly -- of every Madison Avenue creative.

Subliminal Seduction .... Wilson   Bryan   Key, **Prentice-Hall 1973**
Media Sexploitation .... Wilson   Bryan   Key, **Prentice-Hall 1976**

Another controversial book (and series!) that won't go out of print. You are never sure whether Key is telling the truth or wildly stretching the point. Yet his references are impeccable and in the end, while you feel disinclined to go to the end of the line with him, **nevertheless** you stay for most of the journey realizing that he is basically on the right track. Unfortunately, he still lacks a grand theory and in the end what you get out of his books are "how dare they!" **Cigarette Seduction** tells you how to use that information for understanding yourself or getting a better perspective about society in general and the people you know in particular.

Personal Mythology .... Feinstein   &   Krippner, **Tarcher/St. Martin's, 1988**

This is a very interesting book that suffers in the execution. Instead of giving readers a straightforward roadmap to their unique approach of identifying and communicating with **their** personal myth, **the authors** use long-winded and hard-to-follow stories to do it for them. It also spends precious little time dealing with the most fascinating parts of their theories – counter-myths and changing your myth when it no longer serves you. **The book** also neglects to discuss the origin of the personal myth.

The Signs of our Times...................Jack Solomon, Tarcher, 1988

This is the first popular semiotics book written by a practicing semiotician. It skillfully steers a course through the Scylla and Charybdis of the academic community by paying homage to **academia's** heavily Marxist and feminist leanings while staying clear of the "circle of signs" problem. It explains the basis of semiotics as a way of seeing the meaning of everyday objects and ceremonies for what they often are: a system of psychologically perceived conventions arranged and manipulated by the largely patriarchal powers-that-be. Its insights are competent but just that. There is no great psychological depth and nothing on the mythology of human existence. Therefore, it **fails to** provide **a** way of breaking out of that great semiotics bugbear, the "circle of signs" problem**, that is,** the tendency to understand signs in terms of other signs. The semiotician's idea that common sense is really **communal sense**, a silent conspiracy that sustains the interests of the ruling group, is fine but not very helpful to readers who are looking for those fundamental human verities that supersede the eternal relativism of social interpretation.

Cigarette Seduction uses a language of insight that sidesteps the conventional whitewash of societal norms and gives readers a practical use of mythology in their everyday lives. It also shows how that can be used personally to probe the real nature of the people they meet who happen to smoke.

INDIRECTLY RELATED BOOKS
Ashes to Ashes...................Richard Kluger, Random House, 1996
The **'nineties** first big selling book and Pulitzer Prize winner in this field. Marvelously written and researched. Overlong and essentially a business history of Philip Morris.

Smokescreen..........................Philip Hilts, Addison Wesley, 1996
A good "quickie" book that reveals the tobacco industry's dastardly manipulations of congress and, in particular, selling to teens. Basically a business book that hoped to reach an outraged public; unfortunately, they may not be outraged enough to spend $22.

Cigarettes Are Sublime..Richard Klein, Duke University Press, 1995
A popular book that went paperback, but in reality is a scholarly, Barthesian semiotic analysis of smoking based on film and literary sources. Sold to smokers and non smokers alike. Considered by the many in the health movement who have scant affection for the conceit of literature as the work of the antichrist.

Thank You For Smoking.......Chris Buckley, Haperperennial, 1995
A very funny satire on the tobacco debate focusing on a lovable villain: a tobacco industry lobbyist. Moderately popular movie.

GASP!................................**Frank Freudberg, Barricade Books, 1996**
The "Falling Down" and "Network" of cigarette books. A smoker, dying of cancer sets out to take revenge. Fast cut style, bad publisher, and big hopes for a movie.

Understanding Media……..**Marshall McLuhan, McGraw-Hill, 1965**
A breakthrough book that made us understand the multisensory nature of media. **Cigarette Mythology** makes us understand the multisensory nature of everyday living.

Sun Signs………………………..**Linda Goodman, Taplinger, 1968**
Taking the major signs of the Zodiac and attaching each to a quote from **Alice in Wonderland** and **Through the Looking Glass**, Linda Goodman dazzled millions of readers with her penetrating insight. You didn't have to believe in astrology to realize that she was telling the truth about you and the people you knew. But if you didn't believe in astrology she still left the question dangling: How can the stars really influence our lives? How do they **know**, how do they reach us and for heaven's sake, why?

Cigarette Seduction in its own way, answers some of these questions by painting on a much smaller canvas. It doesn't attempt to tell us as much about ourselves but in the end it answers more of those universal questions that arise whenever we start to read between the lines of human nature.

The Official Preppie Handbook…….**Lisa Birnbach, Workman, 1980**
With its insouciance and panache, this book not only described the patrician set by their habits and perennial symbols, but it put semiotics on the map. Yet it never mentioned it by name (it is an ugly and technical word) nor forgot to keep its tongue ever so firmly in cheek so that no one, not even the derided Preppie, could have taken offense.

On the other hand, one could argue, why should they? It was obvious that Birnbach secretly admired preppies and wanted to be one if she wasn't already. Besides which, it is much easier to laugh at yourself when you also happen to own most of everything.

Cigarette Seduction runs a touch deeper and won't create as much laughter in the executive suites of cigarette companies. But it could make smokers and non-smokers alike have a good laugh when they realize how much of the mystique of smoking it manages to uncover. After all, revelation always starts out by appearing to be shocking, then it moves over to the comedy circuit, and ends up in the op-ed pages of the New York Times.

NEWSPAPER AND MAGAZINE ARTICLES OF RELATED INTER-EST:

What About Teen Withdrawal......Alan Brody, July, 1997, Gannett Suburban Newspapers

Boys to Men........................John Leo, US News, June 3, 1997

Uncle Sam No Match for the **Marlboro** Man..... Stewart Elliot, New York Times, September 23, 1997

Verdict Doesn't Faze Philip Morris (Cipallone vs. Lorillard) Newsday (special), June 21, 1988

Pushing Cigarettes Overseas.............................. New York Times Magazine **(Cover Story)** -- July10, 1988

Do Sex and Violence Sell Cigarettes?..........Spy Magazine, August 1988

Personal Mythology...Psychology Today **(Cover Issue)** December 1988

Personal Myths Bring Cohesion to the Chaos of Each Life (The mythical image can offer a script that predicts behavior or signals self-destructive patterns) The New York Times, May 24, 1988

The Big Idea (The **Marlboro** Story)................Advertising Age special issue, November 9th, 1988,

Philip Morris' Big Bite.......New York Times Magazine, April 9, 1989

Source Information

This book is a product of extensive research and was originally presented as a paper before 1984 Popular Culture Association Convention in Toronto, Canada. The presentation took the small gathering of academics by storm and, before long, press photographers and TV cameras were on hand to taking shots of the author holding up his chart of filter types, explaining the *meaning of cigarette filters!*

While this book employs many of the basic techniques and attitudes of semiotics - the interdisciplinary study of signs and the structure of symbolic communication – it **also** adds three key elements: Though the author is not a therapist it makes use of psychoanalytical thinking; it refers to the published writings of well-known researchers in the advertising industry; **and** it shows that products are not only psychologically meaningful but their symbolism is connected with the ancient mythology and mystic rituals of the human race. These are either deliberately worked into the development of the product and its image by the marketer or spontaneously introduced by the consumers, in effect, as an intuitive form of communion with an unconscious force that effectively continues the mythic side of life in a disguised form.

Printed in Great Britain
by Amazon

50391517R00102